FERTILITY
&
Conception

FERTILITY
&
Conception

*The essential guide to boosting
your fertility and conceiving
a healthy baby — from learning
your fertility signals to
adopting a healthier lifestyle*

DR KAREN TREWINNARD

CARROLL & BROWN PUBLISHERS LIMITED

This edition published in 2003 in the United Kingdom by
Carroll & Brown Publishers Limited
20 Lonsdale Road
London NW6 6RD

Previously published in 1999 in the United Kingdom by Ward Lock
A CIP catalogue record for this book is available from the British Library.
ISBN 978-1-903258-63-7
1098765

REPRODUCED BY COLOURSCAN, SINGAPORE
PRINTED AND BOUND IN HONG KONG BY PRINTING EXPRESS

CONTENTS

INTRODUCTION

When my husband and I decided to start a family 21 years ago, no one suggested
that I could prepare myself for conception. In fact, doctors and parents alike
believed that the best way to help a woman have a healthy baby and pregnancy was
to provide her with good antenatal care from about the 12th week of pregnancy.
So, when I was expecting my first daughter I just prayed she would be healthy and
that my dreadful morning, noon, and night sickness would soon stop. By the time I
had my first prenatal check-up, I realised my newly conceived baby was already
fully formed and development from that stage was mostly a matter of growth. But I
had a nagging feeling that I could have done more to prepare myself for the
miraculous event of pregnancy.

Before my next baby – our son – was conceived, I decided to investigate whether a
woman's health before pregnancy could affect its outcome. Although very little
research had been conducted on preconception care programmes, I was amazed at
my findings – the medical journals carried plenty of evidence that factors such as
low body weight or paternal smoking could increase the risk of miscarriage or of
giving birth to an underweight baby. I had been
underweight at the time of my daughter's conception and I now believe this made me prone to
morning sickness. My body was struggling to cope
with the demands of pregnancy and had little in
the way of reserve.

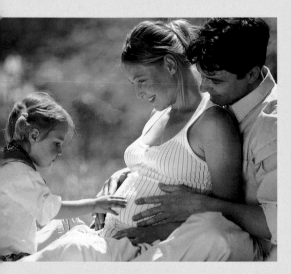

When I became pregnant for the second time, my
weight was normal and I made sure my diet was
full of vitamins. I felt so much better during
that pregnancy, was hardly sick at all, and
my son was born healthy and full of energy.

I have since had two more children and my 20 years' experience as a doctor has ranged from dealing with tiny babies in special care units to treating women in a variety of gynaecology and family planning clinics, many of whom are hoping to conceive. Despite the medical advances in treating infertility, a natural conception is still far more likely to result in a successful pregnancy. I frequently see couples with fertility problems who have been helped to conceive by simply improving their general health rather than expensive and stressful fertility treatments. Of course no one can guarantee that you will instantly conceive and produce a perfect baby, but even while your future baby is still just a longing or merely a twinkle in your eye, you and your partner can both be taking steps toward a healthy conception.

This book will help you understand the marvellous process of fertility in men and women, the miraculous events of conception, and the first weeks of a baby's development. It is full of practical advice covering every area of your health – from the optimum diet to reducing your stress levels – so that you can produce healthier sperm and ova, provide a safe and nurturing environment in utero, and ensure your baby has the best start in life.

I am thrilled that you have taken the time to pick up this book because by taking care of your health before conception, you and your partner are no longer leaving your baby's health in the hands of fate. Congratulations on believing that you can make a difference…and now read on!

DR. KAREN TREWINNARD, B.M. M.F.F.P.

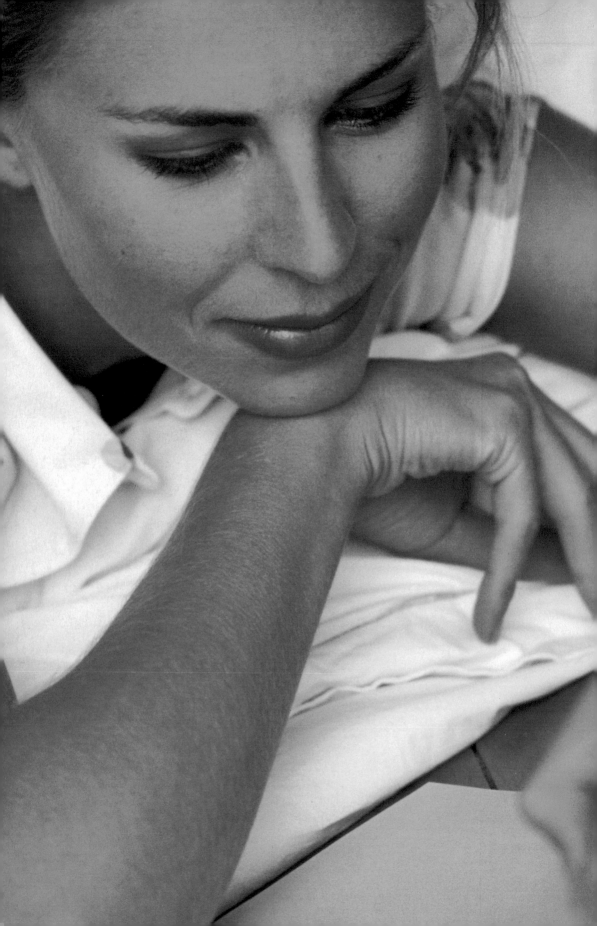

PART I

UNDERSTANDING YOUR FERTILITY

From the moment of conception you were unique. Every human life starts from just one cell formed by a father's sperm and a mother's ovum. Your sex was determined at fertilisation and within days your own reproductive system was developing. Even before you were born your body was equipping you for conception. Understanding how your reproductive system works will help you to appreciate how important your health is before conception — not only to boost your fertility, but also to give your baby the best start in life.

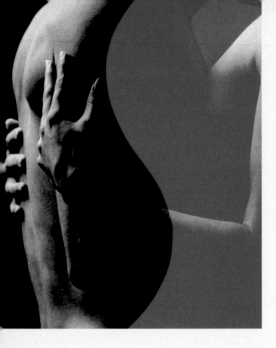

The Fertile Body

It seems amazing but, as a woman, part of you existed inside your grandmother's uterus! Unlike boys, who don't start producing sperm until puberty, girls develop eggs (ova) long before their own birth. This means that the egg (ovum) which eventually united with your father's sperm to create you was already developing when your mother was still growing inside her mother. Indeed, conceiving, carrying and giving birth are probably the most miraculous of all functions the female body can perform.

In the beginning – future mothers

As early as three weeks after you were conceived, your ovaries began to develop and contained about 100 germ cells ready for egg production. Three months before you were born, your tiny ovaries were the scene of frenzied activity as they produced millions of primitive egg cells, called oocytes. By the sixth month of your gestation, about seven million oocytes had formed. By the time you were born, your ovaries contained all the ova you will ever produce throughout your life.

Each tiny oocyte is surrounded by its own set of hormone-producing cells, known as granulosa cells. Together the oocyte and its granulosa cells form a potential chemical factory known as a primordial follicle. At birth, your ovaries contained millions of these basic production units, each of which was capable of maturing and releasing one fertile egg after puberty during a menstrual cycle.

In the years leading up to puberty many of these primordial follicles broke up and were reabsorbed by your body. As you reached puberty, mere thousands remained, lying dormant like seeds in the ground during winter. As an adult in your fertile years, one mature ovum will usually be released each month, ready for fertilisation. In total, you may release around 400 ova during your reproductive life.

In the beginning – future fathers

In contrast to girls, boys don't start manufacturing sperm until puberty. From that time, the testes become busy producing thousands of tiny sperm by the hour. Cells lining half a mile of tubules coiled in the testes divide to produce tiny primitive spermatogonia or sperm-producing cells. The spermatogonia then begin a three-month journey, during which they are transformed into mature, mobile sperm, each one capable of fertilising an ovum to create a new human life.

Because sperm take this long to mature, a man's health is vitally important during the three months before conception. Paying attention to your health during this time will not only improve your fertility, it will also give your future children a better chance of good health.

The fertile woman

A woman's body is beautifully designed to fulfil its role in responding to and giving sexual pleasure, receiving sperm, and providing the ideal environment for sperm to meet and fertilise the ovum she produces each month. It then adapts perfectly to protect, nurture and give birth to her developing child.

At the heart of her body's design are the ovaries that release the ova each month and vital hormones that prime and regulate the reproductive organs. The Fallopian tubes, uterus, cervix and vagina are the other parts of her system.

The ovaries

Each roughly the size of a ripe apricot, the two ovaries produce the ova that carry unique genetic material from the mother (see page 18), which will unite with sperm to create new life. The ovaries are found on either side of the uterus, deep within your pelvis. Each is surrounded by the ends of a Fallopian tube, called the fimbriae. When an ovum is released from one of the ovaries, the hovering fimbriae draw it into the Fallopian tube to await fertilisation.

In addition to releasing an ovum once a month, the ovaries also release oestrogen and progesterone. These two female sex hormones work together to play an important role in the timing of events in a woman's fertility cycle and preparing the reproductive organs for their function at every stage (see page 14).

The amazing ovum

The human egg has two purposes: to carry half the genetic material necessary to create a new individual (the other half is provided by the father's sperm); and to provide all the energy and cellular material necessary to sustain embry-

DID YOU KNOW?

Humans are one of the few mammals that tend to release a single ovum at ovulation to produce a single offspring. With elephants, for example, four ovulations need to take place for there to be enough progesterone for a successful pregnancy. the American nine-banded armadillo, however, can produce four babies from only one ovulation, making identical armadillo quads the norm.

onic development up to a week after fertilisation. This may explain why the egg, at about one-tenth the size of the full stop at the end of this sentence, is the largest cell in the female body.

The Fallopian tubes

Named after the Italian anatomist, Gabriel Fallopus, the Fallopian tubes run from close to each ovary to the uterus, where they open into its top corners. Each tube is about 10 centimetres (4 inches) long and although it looks about the thickness of a drinking straw, the internal canal is only one millimetre ($\frac{1}{25}$ of an inch) wide. The walls surrounding the Fallopian tubes are thick and contain muscle and mucus-secreting glands. The tubes are lined with a carpet of cilia or hairs, which waft the eggs along.

The uterus

A hollow, muscular organ, the uterus is about the size and shape of an upside-down pear. Its thick walls can expand an incredible amount, allowing it to accommodate a growing baby and its placenta during the nine months of pregnancy. By the time a woman is ready to give birth, her uterus is holding not only a full-term baby weighing between 3 and $4\frac{1}{2}$ kilograms (seven and ten pounds), but also the placenta, which is 400 grams (just under a pound) and more than two litres (about half a gallon) of amniotic fluid.

The cervix

The main entrance and exit to the uterus is the cervix, which dips into the upper end of the vagina. The cervix is an amazingly dynamic structure that constantly changes in response to reproductive hormones: it provides a channel through which semen enters the uterus during sexual intercourse; it forms an impenetrable protective barrier when pregnancy occurs; and it is later transformed into a thin sleeve through which the baby's head can slip unimpeded during childbirth. Glands which line and cover the surface of the cervix have a vital role to play in the fertility cycle. They secrete mucus which helps nourish and transport sperm on their journey towards an ovum (see chapter 3: Learning Fertility Awareness).

The vagina

An elastic, muscular tube, the vagina lies between the bladder and the rectum and extends from the cervix to the outside of the body. The

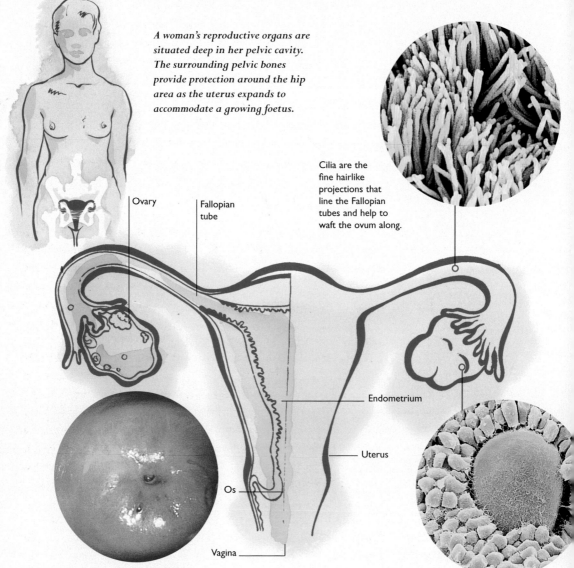

A woman's reproductive organs are situated deep in her pelvic cavity. The surrounding pelvic bones provide protection around the hip area as the uterus expands to accommodate a growing foetus.

Ovary

Fallopian tube

Cilia are the fine hairlike projections that line the Fallopian tubes and help to waft the ovum along.

Endometrium

Uterus

Os

Vagina

The cervix is the gateway to the uterus. It has a tiny dimple — the os — at its centre, which allows menstrual blood to flow out from the uterus and sperm to enter it.

Egg follicles develop inside the ovaries until one has matured and is released into one of the Fallopian tubes.

entrance to the vagina lies between the thick lips of the vulva. The vagina is surrounded by a supporting sling of muscles and its walls are lined with lubricative glands. Their secretions ease the entry of the penis into the vagina during intercourse. The vagina's other functions are to carry menstrual fluids away from the uterus and to expand to form part of the birth canal during labour.

Chemical control of the fertility cycle

An essential part of the female reproductive system is the control centre at the base of the brain. This consists of the hypothalamus and pituitary glands, which secrete vital hormones or chemical messengers that regulate many of the reproductive organs' activities. Together, the hypothalamus, pituitary and ovaries operate a feedback mechanism that synchronises the timing of events in the fertility cycle. This mechanism is dependent on hormone levels in the body. For example, oestrogen produced by the ovaries affects hormone production from another gland, such as the hypothalamus; in effect it switches it on or off. The hormone production of each gland is controlled by feedback information received by chemical messengers from the other glands in the system. This not only ensures that a fertile egg is produced and transported ready for fertilisation, but also that the other events of the menstrual cycle coordinate precisely with ovum production (see also box on page 16).

Unfolding fertility As puberty approached, your pituitary and hypothalamus glands became sensitive to gently increasing amounts of two potent hormones: luteinising hormone (LH) and follicle stimulating hormone (FSH). These hormones, which regulate the menstrual cycle, are sent from the pituitary gland at the base of the brain through the bloodstream to the ovaries. Close by, in the brain, the hypothalamus regulates the pituitary, telling it when to release FSH

CHANGING TIMES

Women today consider it normal to experience a period every month, but in Victorian times, our great, great grandmothers may have had as few as a dozen periods in their entire lifetime. Victorian women often started their large families soon after their first periods at the age of 15 or 16. With nine months for each pregnancy and two to three years spent breast-feeding each baby, they easily could have had only one period every three or four years over the 30 to 35 years of potential fertile life. This is still the case today in those traditional societies where women have children at a young age and breast-feeding is the only form of contraception.

and LH, using information received from the ovaries and other parts of the brain. The pituitary and hypothalamus also regulate other body functions by secreting growth hormone, thyroid stimulating hormone, and the vital hormone that controls the adrenal glands (these sit on top of each kidney and are the body's response centre for physical stress and illness). All these hormones acted rapidly in late childhood to produce the changes associated with puberty, such as the growth spurt and breast development, which heralded your change from girl to woman.

As rising levels of LH and FSH began to circulate in the bloodstream, the primordial follicles containing oocytes (egg cells) were stimulated to mature, and the surrounding granulosa cells started pouring out ever-increasing amounts of oestrogen. During puberty, the ovaries' production of oestrogen might have been a little variable and some of those unpredictable adolescent mood swings may well have been due to changing hormone levels. Before your first period, oestrogen levels built up slowly, but a few months after your first menstrual period a more regular cycle formed. After this, oestrogen and progesterone set the stage each month for fertilisation and successful implantation of an embryo into the uterus.

The hypothalamus and pituitary glands play a vital role in promoting fertility throughout your reproductive years until menopause. As the menopause approaches, the number of primordial follicles rapidly decreases as many age and die, and, despite the efforts of the pituitary to pour out LH and FSH, the ovaries become less and less responsive. At the menopause no follicles or ova remain and the ovaries shrink to about half their original size.

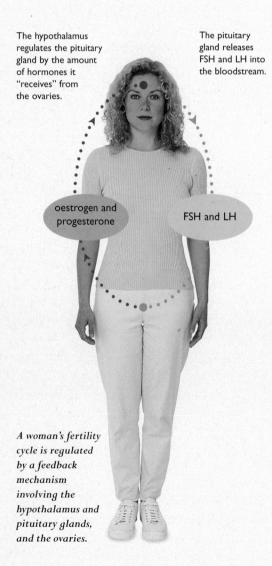

The hypothalamus regulates the pituitary gland by the amount of hormones it "receives" from the ovaries.

The pituitary gland releases FSH and LH into the bloodstream.

oestrogen and progesterone

FSH and LH

A woman's fertility cycle is regulated by a feedback mechanism involving the hypothalamus and pituitary glands, and the ovaries.

Other body changes during puberty As well as the vital changes in the ovaries and uterus, the rest of your body was also affected by new levels of hormones from the pituitary and ovaries. Oestrogen and progesterone stimulated breast development so that your milk glands and ducts began to grow, and this prepared the breast for lactation. Breast development is often quite irregular to start with, and this can cause some girls to experience lumpy and unequal breasts during the early days of puberty. Breasts are often not fully mature until several years after a girl's first menstrual period.

Fat also was laid down during puberty and deposited in all the familiar female places, such as around your hips and thighs. It, too, signalled your emerging fertility and it now accounts for most of the difference in breast size between you and other women. Fat is vital to your fertility. Before you can start to menstruate you need to have reached the crucial weight of about 48 kilograms (106 pounds or 7 stone), regardless of your age or height. You also need to carry a certain amount of fat to act as a reservoir for female hormones. Weight loss, therefore, can be a danger to fertility (see page 101).

Making sense of your menstrual cycle

Roughly once a month during your fertile years, a series of synchronised events prepares your body for pregnancy. Each month an egg ripens in one of your ovaries and is released into the Fallopian tube – an event known as ovulation. Before ovulation, your ovaries produce increasing amounts of oestrogen. This hormone stimulates the lining of the uterus, called the endometrium, to thicken so that it can receive the egg – should it be fertilised. The period of endometrial growth leading up to ovulation is known as the proliferative phase. This phase starts the regrowth of the endometrium (which was shed during the last menstrual period); the glands in the endometrium lengthen and the blood vessels grow.

Natural ways to beat premenstrual syndrome (PMS)

With all the hormonal changes taking place in their bodies each month, it's hardly surprising that 80 per cent of women notice some physical and emotional change during the premenstrual fortnight. Some are positive, such as increased energy, but others, such as irritability, forgetfulness, backache, breast tenderness, headache, fatigue and sweet cravings can make this a difficult time.

Although there are various medical treatments for PMS, most women can alleviate PMS symptoms by simply improving their diet and lifestyle. This is especially useful when you are preparing for pregnancy and want to avoid unnecessary medication that could affect your fertility or harm your unborn baby. To alleviate some of the symptoms of PMS try some of the following:

- Never miss a meal.
- Eat unrefined starchy snacks (such as bananas or rice cakes) every two or three hours. These will keep your blood sugar levels steady and help to stop irritability.
- Cut down on animal fats. A low-fat diet can dramatically improve breast tenderness in three to six months.
- Take a daily walk or do some low impact exercise. Regular exercise boosts your body's natural opiate levels, which helps you to relax and relieves any physical pain.
- Cut down on tea, coffee and cola as the caffeine in these can make you feel more irritable. Try drinking herb and fruit teas instead.
- Take 50–100 microgram doses of Vitamin B6 daily. This seems to help some women, although the effects can wear off after a few months.
- Take 1–3 grams of evening primrose oil supplements daily. Evening primrose oil contains an essential fatty acid, known as gamma linolenic acid (GLA), which helps to ease premenstrual breast tenderness. The benefits usually take a few months to appear, so persevere.

As FSH from the pituitary gland begins to reach the ovaries in increasing amounts, many ovarian follicles are stimulated and start to grow. After a few days, one follicle begins to become dominant and grows to a fluid-filled bubble about 2 cm (an inch) across, on the surface of the ovary. Inside this bubble is the ovum, ready to be released. The fimbriae, the finger-like ends of the Fallopian tube, hover over the follicle.

Once ovulation occurs, the fimbriae sweep the ovum into the Fallopian tube, where it circulates gently in the surrounding fluid, waiting to be fertilised. The ovum can survive in this fluid for between 12 and 24 hours. If fertilisation does not occur, the ovum dies and is shed with the thickened endometrium during menstruation.

As soon as the ovum is released, the follicle reseals itself and becomes a vital unit called the corpus luteum. Latin for "yellow body," the corpus luteum is so named because it looks like a small yellow scar on the surface of the ovary. Once formed, it immediately starts producing progesterone, as well as oestrogen. Together, these hormones prepare the uterus to receive the ovum – should it be fertilised. This is what is known as the secretory phase of the menstrual cycle.

As the endometrium enters the secretory phase, it thickens further and its glands start secreting nourishing fluid. The blood vessels in the endometrium also become longer and more coiled. Should the ovum be fertilised, the corpus luteum will keep on producing progesterone and the thick, secretory endometrium will be able to

WHAT CAUSES OVULATION?

The signal for an ovum to be released during each menstrual cycle is the sudden surge in the pituitary gland's output of luteinising hormone (LH). As the level of oestrogen increases, the hypothalamus gland sends a hormone (luteinising hormone releasing hormone or LHRH) to the pituitary, stimulating the release of large amounts of LH. This travels in the bloodstream to the ovaries, indicating that all is ready for ovulation. The surge of LH in the bloodstream causes the most mature and dominant follicle to release its ovum.

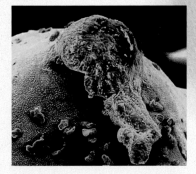

LH stimulates the ovary, which has been primed by FSH, to release a mature ovum.

One follicle starts maturing

Week 2

Mature follicle releases an ovum

Week 1

Week 3

Follicles start developing

Week 4

Corpus luteum starts to form

Corpus luteum shrivels up

The first hormone to peak in the menstrual cycle is oestrogen. This is followed shortly afterwards by LH and a smaller peak of FSH. After ovulation there is a surge of progesterone.

Luteinising hormone (LH)

Follicle stimulating hormone (FSH)

Oestrogen

Progesterone

Week 1   Week 2   Week 3   Week 4

protect and nourish the developing embryo in one of its glands.

If fertilisation does not occur, the corpus luteum will shrivel up and the production of progesterone falls. As a result, the endometrium will begin to shrink and the blood vessels will be compressed. The blood supply is thus decreased, and the thick endometrium dies and will be shed as the menstrual period. The normal menstrual loss a woman experiences varies from a table-spoon to a cupful, and is made up of blood, tissue and mucus.

Lengths of cycle Your menstrual cycle is counted from the day you first begin bleeding until the start of your next period. Although many women have a period every 28 days, the average monthly cycle can be as short as 25 days or as long as 35 days, without there being any abnormality or loss of fertility. The time between ovulation and menstruation (known as the luteal phase) is fixed at around 14 days. This is due to the corpus luteum having a limited life span of 12 to 16 days from the time it is formed after ovulation. However, the build up to ovula-tion can be longer or shorter than the usual 14 days, and this is where most women's cycles vary in length.

As the corpus luteum nears the end of its two-week life span, when menstruation approaches, its production of oestrogen and progesterone falls. The hypothalamus senses this fall soon after menstruation and starts to stimu-late the pituitary again. The pituitary responds by sending out FSH to stimulate the ovaries and your cycle starts all over again.

Because your menstrual cycle depends upon a constant feedback of hormones, anything that affects this can affect your fertility. For example, breast-feeding will inhibit hormone production from the pituitary gland (see page 50), and stress

DID YOU KNOW?

The combined contraceptive pill works by ensuring there are constant levels of proges-terone and oestrogen in the body. The hypothalamus is "tricked" into behaving as if ovulation has already occurred, so that the level of LH from the pituitary never rises high enough to cause ovulation.

or sudden weight loss can also interfere with the hormone pro-duction from the hypothalamus gland (see page 101). On the other hand, simple fertility drugs work by boosting or imitating this hor-monal feedback system to give your ovaries the "kickstart" they require (see page 14).

Changes in cervical mucus
While an ovary is producing an ovum during the first half of the menstrual cycle, the rest of your reproductive system also is responding to the rising levels of oestrogen. These changes provide sperm with the best conditions in which to travel up the Fallopian tubes and fertilise the ovum waiting there. As the ovarian follicles develop and secrete increasing amounts of oestrogen, the cervix responds by producing clear, stretchy mucus.

This cervical mucus is like liquid crystal and is the vital transport medium for sperm. At ovu-lation the mucus provides clear channels – like smooth-sided toboggan runs – for sperm to travel through. The mucus is also energy-rich and nourishing and sperm can survive in the crevices containing the mucus-secreting glands for up to five days prior to ovulation. This means that conception can take place several days after you have had intercourse.

Once through the cervix, the sperm are helped on their journey up to the Fallopian tubes by secretions from the uterus.

After ovulation, progesterone causes the cervical mucus to become thick and sticky. As a result, any sperm approaching the cervix will find their way blocked – the mucus being more like a dense snowdrift than a pathway – and will be unable to pass through. This mucus barrier also protects the uterus and any developing embryo from infection. The changing consisten-

GENES AND CHROMOSOMES

Every human being has a unique set of inherited blueprints, or genes, which is identical in every cell of the body, except the sex cells (sperm and ova). Your genes are like chemical instruction programs within the nucleus or command centre of each cell. Groups of genes determine every characteristic of your body, such as hair and eye colour and the shape and size of your nose. But as well as being responsible for external features, these genetic instructions also program every other tiny detail of human development, such as which cells become bone, which will produce blood cells, and which develop into the nervous system. Genes also control the production of all the hormones and enzymes that allow your body to function from minute to minute – to think, digest food, grow and repair damaged tissue.

Each gene contains a set of instructions (made up of thousands of proteins) for the production of one vital chemical. Thousands of sets of these are filed in the cell nucleus in thread-like structures known as chromosomes, much like files on a computer disk. There are 46 chromosomes in each cell, arranged in 23 pairs, one of each pair coming from the mother and the other from the father.

Usually when cells divide to replace themselves for growth or repair, exact replicas are produced containing the same chromosomes and genes. If you cut your fingertip, your fingerprint will be exactly the same as before when the injury has healed. This process of duplicate cell division is called mitosis. But, the sex cells are produced differently in a unique way called meiosis. This two-stage process first mixes the genes on the chromosomes (to produce a unique combination of genes) and then divides up the chromosome pairs so that the new ovum or sperm contains only 23 single chromosomes, each of which is different from its parent's chromosomes. When two sets of 23 chromosomes (one from a sperm, one from an ovum) fuse at fertilisation, a new individual is created, complete with the normal 46 chromosomes.

THE PROCESS OF MEIOSIS

1. Chromosomes before meiosis. (Only 1 of the 23 pairs of chromosomes found in cells is shown here.)

2. Chromosomes make copies of themselves. The copies are called chromatids. Each of the double chromosomes then pairs up with its partner. A pair of double chromosomes is shown.

3. The chromatids start to exchange blocks of genes so each double chromosome now contains a unique set of genes.

4. The chromosome pairs then separate to opposite ends of the nucleus, ready for the cell to divide.

5. The first division is completed and the 2 new cells each contain 23 double chromosomes (only 1 double in each new cell is shown here).

6. At ovulation the second division begins and the double chromosomes split and start to separate. The separation finishes at fertilisation.

7. Each new cell contains 23 single chromosomes (the extra genetic material has been discarded). So, when they unite during conception they will have the necessary 23 pairs.

cy of cervical mucus is one of the best indications of when you are likely to be most fertile and is explained in greater detail in chapter 3: Learning Fertility Awareness.

The fertile man

Men, unlike women, can be fertile every day of their adult lives. As well as the daily manufacture, storage, and transport of sperm, a man's reproductive system has to deliver the sperm into a woman's vagina and produce male sex hor-

mones. The primary male sex organs are the two testes (the female equivalent of the ovaries) and the penis, but the prostate gland and Cowper's (bulbourethral) glands also play an important role in male fertility.

The testes

These two oval-shaped organs lie in a pouch of skin outside the body called the scrotum. Here the testes are kept cool, unlike the ovaries which are inside a woman's body. Each testicle consists of hundreds of tiny, tightly coiled tubes called

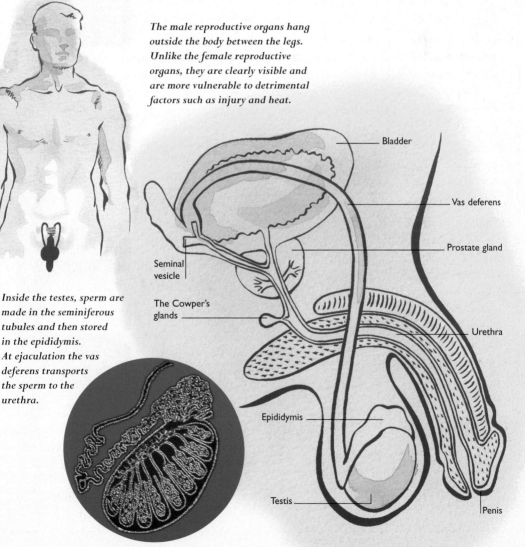

The male reproductive organs hang outside the body between the legs. Unlike the female reproductive organs, they are clearly visible and are more vulnerable to detrimental factors such as injury and heat.

Inside the testes, sperm are made in the seminiferous tubules and then stored in the epididymis. At ejaculation the vas deferens transports the sperm to the urethra.

Bladder

Vas deferens

Prostate gland

Seminal vesicle

The Cowper's glands

Urethra

Epididymis

Testis

Penis

seminiferous tubules and it is here that thousands of sperm are manufactured every minute after puberty. Scattered between the seminiferous tubules are two vital types of cell: Leydig and Sertoli cells. The Leydig cells are where the male sex hormone testosterone is produced, and the Sertoli cells nourish immature sperm (called spermatids) until they have grown a tail and are ready to move on to the next stage of their journey.

The penis

The penis contains three columns of erectile tissues that are rich in blood vessels. These allow the penis to become erect when a man becomes sexually aroused. The smallest column is called the corpus spongiosum. It surrounds the urethra and extends to the tip of the penis to form the glans, the most sensitive part of the penis. The two other columns form the corpus cavernosa. These

DID YOU KNOW?

In the time of the 18th-century German composer, Bach, choirboys were expected to lose their soprano voices around the age of 17. However, due to improved diets and better general health, choirboys today are more likely to develop an alto voice around the age of 13.

spongy columns of tissue are much longer than the penis and anchor it firmly to the pelvic floor, the muscular area between the legs that extends from the base of the penis to around the anus.

After a man reaches orgasm, his levels of adrenaline automatically rise and this causes the arteries feeding the spongy tissues in the penis to constrict slightly. This reduces the blood supply to the penis and the penis becomes soft again as the congested veins in the spongy tissues empty. This process is called detumescence. Because adrenaline causes detumescence, stress can cause erectile problems and this is discussed further in chapter 7: Improving Your Physical and Emotional Health.

From each testis, sperm are transported via one long tube – the epididymis and the vas deferens – to the penis. The epididymis is the long, coiled tube lying at the back of each testis, and is formed by all the tiny seminiferous tubules from the testis joining together. Sperm from each testis travel along each epididymis and pass into the vas deferens. These are the tubes you can feel just beneath the loose skin at the top of each side of the scrotum. Each vas deferens is about 46 cm (18 inches) long and transfers sperm to the prostate gland, on their way to being ejaculated.

When a man becomes sexually aroused, blood collects in the tissues of his penis and it becomes engorged and erect. This enables it to penetrate the vagina so that sperm can be ejaculated near the cervix.

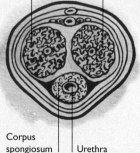

Corpus
cavernosa

Corpus
spongiosum | Urethra

Three columns of spongy tissue in the penis (seen left as a cross section) allow it to become erect.

How sperm are produced

While egg production in a woman begins before she is even born (see page 10), spermatogonia (the primitive sperm-producing cells) lie dormant in the testes throughout childhood, and start to mature only at the time of puberty to become spermatocytes.

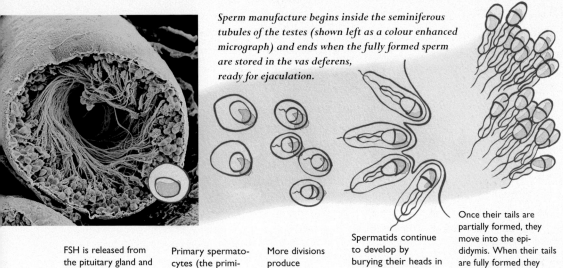

Sperm manufacture begins inside the seminiferous tubules of the testes (shown left as a colour enhanced micrograph) and ends when the fully formed sperm are stored in the vas deferens, ready for ejaculation.

FSH is released from the pituitary gland and triggers sperm production in the testes.

Primary spermatocytes (the primitive sperm cells) start to replicate by meiosis.

More divisions produce young sperm, called spermatids.

Spermatids continue to develop by burying their heads in Sertoli cells, where they receive nourishment.

Once their tails are partially formed, they move into the epididymis. When their tails are fully formed they swim up into the vas deferens and are called spermatozoa.

The production of sperm is triggered by LH and FSH – the same hormones that initiate sexual maturity in girls. As levels of LH from the pituitary gland in the brain rose in puberty, specialised Leydig cells in the testes started to produce a constant supply of the male hormone, testosterone.

As well as promoting the production of viable sperm, testosterone controls muscle growth and other bodily changes during puberty. It also affects male libido, regulates the growth of the prostate gland, and controls the secretions of prostatic and seminal fluid. A young man usually becomes fertile soon after his main adolescent growth spurt when his voice breaks, pubic hair grows, his penis and testes grow, and he begins to ejaculate. This may be some time before he reaches his adult height and the male features of facial and body hair develop fully.

Under the control of the hypothalamus in the brain, the pituitary releases FSH, which stimulates the spermatocytes in the testes to start replicating themselves by meiosis (see page 18). The resulting cells (called secondary spermatocytes) then divide and produce young sperm, known as spermatids.

Round and tailless, spermatids bear little resemblance to the familiar tadpole shape of mature sperm. As they continue to develop, they bury their heads in specialised supporting cells known as Sertoli cells, which provide all the nourishment sperm need to mature. Once their tails are partially formed, the sperm move into the epididymis, the coiled mass of tubes lying on top of the testes. In the weeks that sperm are stored there, their tails finish growing and they start to swim. Now fully motile, they pass into the vas deferens where the maturation process is completed. At about 46 cm (18 inches) long, each vas deferens has an enormous storage capacity (after a vasectomy, it can take up to 30 ejaculations before all remaining sperm are expelled). The sperm are kept in the vas deferens until they are ejaculated through the erect penis during orgasm.

Consisting of three parts, sperm are ideally suited to their task of carrying genetic material to a female egg. The head contains the nucleus, where the 23 chromosomes are stored in compact form, and the acrosome tip, which helps the sperm to penetrate the egg. The long tail propels the sperm forwards at a rate of about

3 millimetres (an eighth of an inch) every minute.

The manufacture, maturation, storage, and eventual ejaculation of sperm takes between 70 and 100 days. It is during these three months that sperm are particularly vulnerable to damage from viruses and toxins caused by smoking and x-rays. And because sperm carry half the genetic material necessary to create a new life, it's just as vital for men as it is for women to look after their health before conception. With all the division and rearrangement of genetic material that happens during sperm production, it's easy to see how genetic mistakes could occur. What is amazing, however, is that the majority of sperm are produced without any genetic defect.

Semen: a sperm's survival kit

Sperm are not ejaculated from the body on their own but are released during orgasm in a milky fluid called semen or seminal fluid.

As well as sperm, semen is made up of secretions from two specialised glands, the prostate and Cowper's glands, and fluid from the seminal vesicles. There are hundreds of substances present in healthy semen, and although the function of many of these is not yet understood, they all seem to have a role in keeping the sperm viable, well nourished and energised so they can reach the Fallopian tube where an ovum may be waiting to be fertilised.

Semen from one ejaculation is usually 2–5 millilitres (about a teaspoon) in volume, and has a whitish–grey colour. Immediately after ejaculation the semen is fairly thick, but after a few minutes it liquefies and releases more sperm into

DID YOU KNOW?

Because sperm and ova are invisible to the naked eye, early scientists and philosophers thought a baby resulted from a man planting his "seed" in a woman. It was not until 1678, after the invention of the microscope, that the existence of sperm was discovered by Dutch scientist Anton van Leeuwenhoek (the ovum had to wait another 150 years to be identified). However, van Leeu-wenhoek mistakenly thought that the head of a sperm carried a baby in miniature form, which was delivered into the mother for nurturing via the semen.

the female reproductive tract. Only about 20 per cent of the volume of semen consists of sperm. Around 70 per cent of the fluid is supplied by the seminal vesicles and the remaining 10 per cent comes from the prostate and Cowper's glands.

The seminal vesicles These lie behind the bladder and secrete fluid into the ejaculatory ducts. They are important because they provide two substances vital for fertility: sugars (mostly fructose), which are a ready source of energy for the sperm on their arduous journey, and hormones called prostaglandins, which help the sperm to swim and may have an important part to play in helping the ovum and sperm to meet.

Secretions from the seminal vesicles also contain the protein that causes semen to "clot" immediately after ejaculation.

The prostate gland This is about the size of a chestnut, although it tends to grow larger with age. It surrounds the urethra at the base of the bladder and contains approximately 20 ducts that release secretions into the semen.

The prostatic fluid is slightly alkaline, which helps to neutralise the woman's slightly acidic vaginal fluids. It also contains many important enzymes, minerals and proteins. One of these enzymes is responsible for reliquefying the semen.

The Cowper's glands These two pea-sized glands at the base of the penis secrete a small amount of clear fluid into the urethra both before and during ejaculation, as a response to sexual stimulation. The secretions counteract the acids in the urethra and help lubricate the tip of the penis to aid intercourse. They are also known as the bulbourethral glands.

The process of ejaculation

When a man is sexually aroused, messages from his nervous system cause an involuntary reaction – blood rushes into his penis and causes the spongy tissue inside it to expand. As the penis swells up, the veins that usually carry blood away from it are flattened and blocked, trapping the blood in the penis so it becomes rigid and erect. The erection is maintained until ejaculation (the release of semen) or loss of sexual interest.

Like erection, ejaculation is a reflex action. Just before orgasm, a small drop of semen may appear at the tip of the penis. This consists mainly of lubricating fluid from the Cowper's glands, but it can also contain a few sperm. Then, at the height of sexual pleasure, the epididymis contracts and sends the sperm and fluid up into the vas deferens. Secretions from the prostate gland add to the seminal fluid for the first spurt of the ejaculate. The seminal vesicles then contract rhythmically to release fluid that provides most of the volume of the second and subsequent spurts of ejaculate.

While up to five spurts may occur in quick succession during sexual intercourse, the majority of sperm are released in the first spurt. Deposited in the woman's vagina, the sperm are now ready to embark on their long and perilous journey towards the waiting egg. Only a few will succeed in reaching the Fallopian tubes. The obstacles faced by the sperm, and the events of fertilisation, are described in chapter 2: The Process of Conception.

SEX CELL DIFFERENCES

Despite their differences in size (ova are 20 times larger than sperm), the female sex cell and the male sex cell carry the same amount of genetic material required for normal foetal development. In this way, they are just as important as each other for the process of conception.

	SPERM	OVUM
When manufacture begins	Puberty	During prenatal development
Quantities produced	About 1,000 a second or 100 million a day	Several million: about 10,000 are left at puberty
Time from production to release	About 100 days	Up to 50 years
Quantities released	Millions in each ejaculation	Generally one per month
When released	Puberty to old age	Puberty to menopause
Life span	Up to 5 days in the right circumstances	12–24 hours
Size	0.05 mm (0.02 inches) long	0.1 mm (0.004 inches) in diameter
Mobility	Swims 3 mm (⅛ inch) per minute	Unable to move unaided

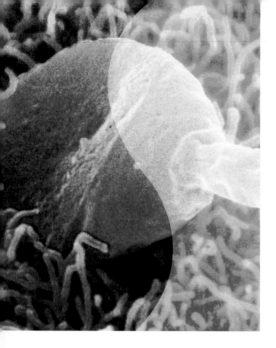

The Process of Conception

Conception is the first stage in a baby's nine-month journey through pregnancy. It begins at the moment of fertilisation – when sperm and ovum unite – and marks the start of a new and unique human life. The process continues until the rapidly dividing ball of cells that forms the tiny embryo implants itself into the protective and nourishing environment of the endometrium lining the uterus.

Fertilisation

When a man ejaculates during sexual intercourse, semen spurts out into the top of his partner's vagina and deposits literally millions of sperm there. This may seem an astonishing number considering just one ovum is waiting to be fertilised, but up to 99 per cent of the semen drains away from the vagina after intercourse. Of the 500 million or so sperm released during each ejaculation, only about 100 survive the journey up through the uterus and Fallopian tubes to meet the waiting ovum. Some sperm may enter the cervix directly after ejaculation, but most start travelling in earnest 5 to 40 minutes after ejaculation, when the semen liquefies after initially clotting.

In the days leading up to ovulation, a woman's cervical mucus forms penetrable swimming channels through the cervix. Prostaglandin hormones in the semen may help the sperm travel towards the site of fertilisation by causing muscle contractions in the uterus and Fallopian tubes, bringing the sperm and ovum closer together. Some sperm may reach the Fallopian tubes within minutes of ejaculation, whereas others take a day or more. This means that sperm are sometimes capable of fertilising an ovum up to five days after a single act of intercourse.

Capacitation

Sperm are being nourished all the time by secretions in the seminal fluid and cervical mucus. For example, one chemical from the epididymis (called carnatine) helps mature the sperm, while the zinc-rich prostatic secretions protect the sperm from infection. Sperm also benefit from certain chemicals in the cervical and uterine fluids, which make it possible for the sperm to penetrate the ovum before actual fertilisation. This process of stimulation is known as capacitation and causes the outer layer of the sperm head (the acrosome tip) to leak some potent enzymes that help to dissolve the membrane surrounding the ovum (called the zona pellucida). Capacitation can also be stimulated in the laboratory to make test-tube fertilisation more successful (see also chapter 11: What Next?).

The point of contact

Once some capacitated sperm make contact with the ovum, their enzymes break down the zona pellucida until one sperm head (containing the 23 chromosomes from the father's gene pool: see page 18) enters the ovum, leaving its tail behind in the process. The penetrating sperm stimulates the ovum to finish the second meiotic division so that 23 single chromosomes from the mother's gene pool appear. At this moment, all other sperm are excluded and the genetic material from the father's sperm and the mother's ovum fuse together to form a new and unique combination. The newly fertilised ovum now contains 46 chromosomes with all the genetic information it needs to divide, grow and develop into a perfectly formed human baby.

CARRYING THE LOAD

Sea horses belong to one of the few species in the animal kingdom where fertilisation takes place in the male body. During the mating process, these tiny creatures coil about each other, belly-to-belly. Within a few seconds, the female sea horse squirts hundreds of her eggs into a pouch on the belly of the male sea horse. The male sea horse's sperm ducts then empty into the pouch and the eggs are quickly fertilised. About two to four weeks later, the male sea horse experiences a series of shuddering contractions and hundreds of baby sea horses shoot out from his pouch.

Implantation

The newly fertilised ovum, now known as a zygote, is wafted down the Fallopian tube towards the uterus by cilia, a carpet of soft, gently moving hairs. The rhythmical movements of the muscles in the walls of the Fallopian tube also help with this process. The zygote starts to replicate itself about 24 to 36 hours after fertilisation and carries on dividing every few hours until it forms a small ball of cells, which is called a morula. The morula arrives in the uterus by about seven days after ovulation. All the while, progesterone secreted by the corpus luteum has been preparing the endometrium to receive the fertilised egg.

Up to 100 capacitated sperm may help to break down the zona pellucida, but only one will penetrate it to fertilise the waiting ovum.

Once the ovum has been fertilised, it rapidly divides into two cells and is called a zygote.

Cell division continues until there is a solid bundle of cells, which is called a morula.

When there are about 100 cells, the egg (now called a blastocyst) buries itself into the endometrium.

At ovulation, a ripe ovum is released from its follicle and drawn into the Fallopian tube.

The journey of the ovum – from the time it is fertilised in the Fallopian tube until it embeds in the lining of the uterus – takes about seven days.

Still dividing every few hours, the morula forms a hollow ball of about 100 cells called a blastocyst. The blastocyst settles on the endometrium and begins to embed itself there. This process, known as implantation, is completed by about seven days after fertilisation and seems to be an active one on the part of the blastocyst, which buries itself safely in the tissues of the endometrium where it can receive a reliable supply of nutrients.

The placenta

After implantation, the blastocyst has to gather its nourishment from the neighbouring cells of its mother and dispose of its waste through them. But over the next few weeks, the outer cells of the blastocyst (now called an embryo) form part of a special organ called the placenta. As the placenta and the embryo's own kidneys and circulation begin to develop, the nutritional and waste exchanges take place on the maternal surface of the placenta.

At first the corpus luteum remains the vital source of hormones sustaining the pregnancy. One of its hormones, progesterone, probably stops the mother's body from rejecting the embryo, which is in fact foreign to her immune system. Similar to the way organ transplant patients are given drugs to suppress their immune systems in order to prevent their bodies from rejecting the donor organ, progesterone may help "blind" the mother's tissues to keep them from recognising the baby and its placenta as foreign.

The placenta not only provides a site for the exchange of the developing baby's nutrients and waste products, it also produces hormones. It starts by secreting human chorionic gonadotrophin (HCG), a hormone that stimulates the corpus luteum to continue producing progesterone. In fact, HCG is produced so early in pregnancy that it forms the basis for most modern pregnancy testing kits (see page 34).

Although the corpus luteum is the initial source of progesterone, if it doesn't receive stimulus from the developing placenta, it would quickly die and a menstrual period would start.

Gradually, over the next ten weeks of pregnancy, the placenta takes over progesterone production and the corpus luteum shrivels up to form a small scar on the surface of the ovary.

The vital first ten weeks

After implantation the embryo develops very quickly. By the time a woman has missed her first period the embryo's nervous system is already beginning to form. Its circulation also develops early and a simple blood-pumping system is in place by the third week of the embryo's life. This rapidly develops into the more sophisticated heart and blood vessels that circulate blood between the baby and the placenta for the exchange of nutrients, waste products, oxygen and carbon dioxide.

Sex: how often is enough?

Despite Nature's apparently foolproof system in which millions of sperm have the opportunity to fertilise an ovum each month, you may find it difficult to conceive if you have sex infrequently. This maybe because the times you choose to make love aren't coinciding with your fertile phase (see also chapter 3: Learning Fertility Awareness).

About seven out of ten couples will conceive within a month if they have sex every day, but only one or two couples will be successful if they have sex just once a week. But if you are aware of your fertility signals, just one carefully timed act of intimacy may be all you need to hit the jackpot!

However, before you embark on a daily baby-making schedule, you should bear in mind that sex too frequently may actually lower your partner's sperm count (not to mention your energy levels)! In this way, it could affect your ability to conceive.

A man's sperm count may fall after ejaculation and rise again after several days of abstinence, although after five days of abstinence sperm may become less mobile and start ageing. For most men, sex every two to three days will give a healthy sperm count and prolonged abstinence is not recommended to raise the sperm count.

You may find it heartening to know that the majority of couples conceive within a year if they have intercourse two or three times a week.

At two weeks the embryo's nervous system is beginning to develop.

At four weeks the primitive organs, such as the liver and lungs, are starting to form.

At six weeks the sex organs (testes or ovaries) begin to develop.

At eight weeks the brain, spinal cord and nerves have formed.

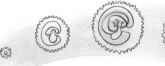
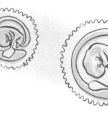

At three weeks the embryo has developed a simple blood-pumping system.

At five weeks limb buds begin to grow and there is a recognisable head and body.

By ten weeks your baby's fingers and toes have formed.

The most important development occurs in the first 10 weeks after fertilisation. After this period, foetal development is mostly a matter of growth.

The third week after fertilisation is also the time when the embryo develops its characteristic C-shape. As well as a head and bottom end, the embryo has a discernible left and right and front and back. A dark stripe down its back curls over to form a groove. In the following week, this seals up to become a neural tube and will later develop into the spinal cord and brain.

Four weeks after fertilisation, two tiny discs of pigment are starting to form on either side of the embryo's head. These are the optic vessels which will develop into your baby's eyes. Inside the body, primitive organs, such as the lungs and liver, are starting to form.

Five weeks after fertilisation, the foetus has a recognisable head, eyes and body. Although there is still a distinct tail, tiny limb buds have started to grow and these will later form arms and legs. The digestive tract is beginning to form and the umbilical cord is developing.

By six weeks, the testes or ovaries are beginning to appear. The limb buds which appeared only a week ago have differentiated into hand and shoulder segments and may be flexed at the elbows and wrists. Eyelids are starting to form over the baby's eyes and external ear structures are starting to develop on the side of the neck. An upper lip and the tip of a nose are also beginning to appear on the face.

By eight weeks, the baby's complete body plan has been laid down. The brain, spinal cord and nerves have formed, and these need only to grow and mature over the months of pregnancy that follow.

Ten weeks after fertilisation, the baby has hands with fingers and feet with toes that it can move and wiggle. All the major internal organs are formed and the external sex organs will look recognisably male or female.

By the third month of pregnancy the baby is fully formed in miniature and looks like a tiny human being. He or she will continue to grow rapidly over the next few months of pregnancy. Human growth is never so fast as it is in these first vital months of life: even the adolescent growth spurt is insignificant compared with the rate at which babies grow in the uterus, where they need the best nourishment and protection to develop healthily.

Is there a best position for intercourse?

To say that Nature is generous with her supply of sperm in a single ejaculate is an understatement. When a woman is fertile, her abundant supply of cervical mucus usually ensures that enough sperm can swim up through the cervix, regardless of which position you choose to make love. The best position is probably the one you and your partner find most enjoyable, as you are likely to be very relaxed. If the semen seems to run out of your vagina after intercourse, don't worry. This occurs naturally as the semen liquefies after clotting and plenty of sperm should have safely embarked on their journey beforehand.

However, if you have a retroverted uterus (that is, tilted backwards instead of forwards), your cervix may not dip into the pool of ejaculate after intercourse. Although sperm should be propelled through the cervix during ejaculation, you can encourage latecomers to swim through by lying on your back after intercourse with a pillow under your pelvis for a while afterwards.

Boy or Girl?

Whether a boy or girl is conceived depends on the chromosomes carried in the sperm. Of the 23 chromosomes in each sperm and ovum, only one determines sex. All girls have a pair of X chromosomes – one from their mother and one from their father – as their sex chromosomes. Boys have one X from their mother and the male or Y chromosome from their father. Therefore, if the sperm fertilising the ovum carries an X chromosome, the resulting embryo will have two X chromosomes (XX) and a girl is conceived. If the sperm carries a Y chromosome, the fertilised cell will have one X and one Y chromosome (XY) and a boy will be conceived.

Couples have tried to influence the sex of their babies for thousands of years and every civilisation has folklore on how to conceive a boy or a girl. For instance, ancient Jewish teachings suggested that if a woman reached

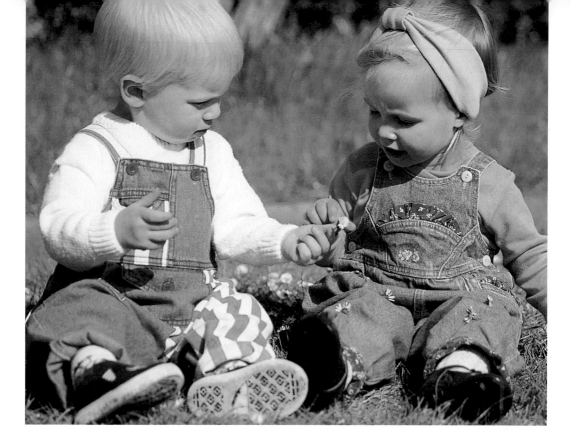

A baby boy gets an X chromosome from his mother and a Y chromosome from his father.

A baby girl gets an X chromosome from her mother and an X chromosome from her father.

orgasm during sexual intercourse before her husband, then she would conceive a male child; "If a woman emits her semen first she bears a male child. If the man emits his semen first she bears a female child." (Babylonian Talmud, tractate Niddah, page 31a.)

As well as folklore, various scientific theories claim to improve the chances of conceiving a child of a particular sex. No method of sex selection is guaranteed, but you can certainly have fun trying! On a more serious note, any couple considering choosing the sex of their child should think carefully about their reaction to conceiving a child of either sex: as no method is guaranteed, be prepared to welcome a son or a daughter (see also page 33).

Current methods of increasing the chances of conceiving a boy or a girl rest on the fact that "male" sperm – those bearing a Y chromosome – are lighter, swim faster, and are less acid-resistant than "female" sperm, which carry an X chromosome. The vagina is slightly acid, but the cervical mucus is alkaline. Cervical mucus secreted several days before ovulation is slightly less alkaline than it normally is when close to ovulation, however, and so may favour female sperm. Because of this, it's been suggested that having intercourse only on the days leading up to ovulation will increase the chance of having a girl. Conversely, to conceive a boy the advice is to make love as close to ovulation as possible, when the fertile cervical mucus is at its peak and more alkaline, therefore benefiting male sperm.

TWINS: TWO FOR THE PRICE OF ONE

Occasionally after the first division, the two cells of a zygote develop into two separate embryos. This results in identical twins – two babies who have the same genetic makeup and are of the same sex.

Non-identical or fraternal twins are conceived when two ova are released from an ovary and both are fertilised by two separate sperm. They aren't necessarily the same sex and are no more alike than any two brothers or sisters from the same parents. Fraternal twins are more common than identical twins, and often run in a family (women can inherit an increased tendency to release more than one egg at ovulation – usually within 12 hours of each other). Fraternal twins have two separate placentas, whereas identical twins share the same placenta.

The chance of conceiving identical twins naturally is about 1 in 80 pregnancies. Twins and other multiple pregnancies are more common after certain forms of fertility treatment that either stimulate the ovaries to release more than one egg per cycle, or where several "test-tube" embryos are replaced in the uterus at once (see also page 185).

Other advice to increase the chances of conceiving a boy or a girl includes douching the vagina with weak vinegar (which is acid) to promote the passage of female sperm in the vagina, or bicarbonate of soda (which is alkaline) to help the passage of male sperm in the vagina. Most doctors, however, don't recommend douching as it can introduce infection into the vagina. Douching is also unlikely to affect the sperm, which come surrounded by nourishing semen. In the US female-favouring acid gels and male-favouring alkaline gels are available commercially and are safer than douching. They can be inserted into the vagina before intercourse using an applicator. It has also been suggested that ejaculating low in the vagina, away from alkaline cervical mucus, may favour the acid-resistant female sperm. But this is unlikely to make a difference as fertile cervical mucus flows right throughout the vagina in any case.

While putting these theories into practice is harmless, there is no good scientific evidence that they work. In 1984, a world-wide survey conducted by the World Health Organisation on the effectiveness of deter-

TIME TO TALK
A son or a daughter?

If you or your partner feel strongly about wanting to have a child of a particular sex, take time to discuss why. Boy or girl, your child will need to feel loved and welcomed for him- or herself, not its gender. Perhaps a man wants a boy to fulfil his lost ambitions or a woman may hope for a close friend in a daughter. If you can't explain to your partner why you so desperately want a son or daughter, try asking each other the following questions – they may be a useful starting point for discussion:

- Do you hope for a son or daughter to share your interests? How will you feel if they don't?
- How did you feel about being a boy or girl when you were little? Were boys and girls treated differently in your family?
- Do you think society favours men or women?
- Do you find boys or girls more appealing? For what reasons?
- Do you think boys or girls are most likely to behave well or succeed academically?

mining a baby's sex through various methods produced conflicting results from regions as varied as New Zealand, Chile and Africa. For example, one study, in Nigeria, claimed a 95 per cent success rate: couples who wanted a son were advised to use the Billings' method to detect the peak day of fertile mucus (see page 47), then to only have intercourse on or after this day, close to ovulation. However, another study in New Zealand found that the opposite was happening and over 60 per cent of babies conceived were girls. Remember, any method has a 50 per cent chance of "working" for you!

Sperm separation techniques

Many people have personal reasons for wanting a daughter or a son, but sometimes there are sound medical reasons for wanting to select the sex of a baby, for example when a child of a particular sex is at risk of inheriting a disease.

The X and Y chromosomes contain not only all the genetic material necessary for the development of female or male sexual characteristics, but also many other genes. In rare cases, genetic defects are carried on the X chromosome. Such defects will have less impact if they are masked by a second, unaffected X chromosome, as in a healthy female. But a Y chromosome is unable to mask an X chromosome, so if a male inherits a defective X chromosome he will be affected by disease. Duchenne muscular dystrophy and some types of haemophilia are hereditary sex-linked disorders; both affect males only, although women who are carriers can pass the gene on to their children.

Couples at risk of having a child with a sex-linked genetic disorder can now seek help from gender clinics. These offer sperm-sorting techniques, whereby filters, dyes and electrical charges help to separate the lighter and more agile Y-bearing sperm from the heavier X sperm. The sperm can then be used for artificial insemination. Nevertheless, even the most sophisticated methods of sperm separation are fallible and success cannot be guaranteed. Sex selection for inherited disorders is backed up by termination. Gender clinics are sometimes attended by couples wanting to choose the sex of their baby for social reasons. However, in the UK this is not within the accepted medical guidelines and termination of a healthy foetus on grounds of sex is still not legal.

Some women claim they know they're pregnant from the very moment of conception. This may be because of intuition or because they notice some symptoms of pregnancy (see below). Others don't experience any symptoms until weeks after they have missed their first period. This is unusual, however, and most women begin to notice common signs of pregnancy a couple of weeks after a missed period.

How can you tell you're pregnant?

Signs of early pregnancy

The first and most reliable sign that a woman is pregnant is when she has missed a period or her period is very light. It's important to remember, however, that periods can be missed for other reasons, such as stress (see page 113). Conversely, some harmless bleeding may occur during early pregnancy.

As early as a week after conception you might feel the urge to urinate more often than usual and this may be taken as a sign of pregnancy. A frequent need to urinate is due to the effects of changing hormonal levels and, later, the pressure of your expanding uterus on your bladder. You may

Can you influence your baby's sex?

Although there is an equal chance of conceiving a boy or a girl, there are some things you can try which may increase your chance one way or the other.

For a girl

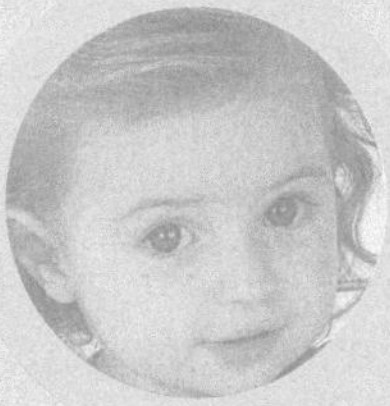

Have intercourse up to two or three days before ovulation

Ejaculate low in the vagina, away from the alkaline cervical mucus

Consider using acidic gel formulated for this purpose

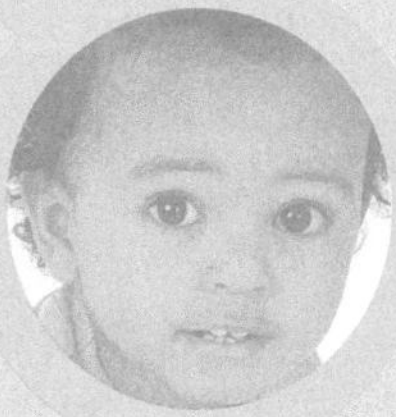

Have intercourse as close to ovulation as possible

Ejaculate high in the vagina, near the alkaline cervical mucus

Consider using alkaline gel formulated for this purpose

For a boy

also feel bloated around the abdomen as a result of water retention. Your breasts may become larger and feel tender, tingly or lumpy. During pregnancy, the veins around the breasts often appear more prominent and the nipples can deepen in colour.

So-called morning sickness is a common sign of pregnancy, but you might also feel sick or hungry at any time of the day or night. This is probably caused by rising levels of the hormones progesterone and HCG. You may also start to have cravings for unusual foods, such as oysters, pickled gherkins or celery, and this may be an indication that you are pregnant. You may suddenly go off drinks, such as coffee, tea or red wine, from early on in pregnancy.

The effects of rising levels of progesterone can also cause unusual tiredness, as well as a change in bowel motions, which could be loose or constipated. A peculiar, metallic taste in the mouth can occur very soon after conception, but usually subsides later in pregnancy.

A woman's intuition

Although a few women may not realise that they are pregnant – even after they have missed a period or two! – other women sense they may be pregnant simply by intuition. Kathy is one of them.

"I remember the precise moment when I realised that I was pregnant with Natasha. My other children, Rachel who was then five, and Ben who had just turned three, were playing a game of hide-and-seek in the typically untidy, but cheerful bedroom they shared.

I had come in with a plate of biscuits and milk and started picking up and tidying away some of their toys. I lay down and stretched out my arm to reach for some books that had slipped under their bunk beds...and woke up about ten minutes later!

As I remembered the all-consuming tiredness that had overwhelmed me in my previous pregnancies, I thought to myself, 'either I'm sick or I'm pregnant.' After that incident, confirming my pregnancy with a test was just a formality!"

Testing for pregnancy

If you have missed a period and are experiencing one or more of the above symptoms, a variety of tests are available that can confirm an early pregnancy. Most of these work by detecting HCG, the pregnancy hormone that is produced by the placenta and appears in the mother's blood and urine from the earliest days of pregnancy.

Although tests do vary in accuracy, many are extremely sensitive and register tiny amounts of HCG even before you even miss your first period. Others will give a positive result only one to two weeks after your missed period (three to four weeks after conception).

Urine tests These rely on the fact that HCG is present in a pregnant woman's urine. Most test kits or solutions contain antibodies to HCG that are chemically attached to a dye or small particles in the solution. If HCG is present, it will bind to the HCG-sensitive antibodies and cause the dye to change colour or the solution to go cloudy as the particles stick together.

Urine tests can be carried out at a doctor's surgery, a pharmacy, or by yourself at home. Their reliability increases the more time passes. For example, most are 90 per cent reliable 10 to 14 days after a missed period. Some over-the-counter tests are more sensitive and can detect a pregnancy earlier. Because urine is highly concentrated first thing in the morning it's best to test the first urine you pass (called early morning urine or EMU). If you work night shifts or get disturbed during the night, make sure the sample of urine you test is collected after you've had your main sleep.

Blood tests Performed by a doctor, these definitive tests can detect small amounts of HCG in maternal blood as early as eight to ten days after conception. A woman's blood is usually only tested if her urine tests are not giving a definite answer. Her blood may also be tested if there is an urgent need to confirm a pregnancy, for instance, if an ectopic pregnancy (see page 158) is suspected. Bear in mind, however, that HCG levels drop only gradually after miscarriage or termination, and may cause a false positive result. A repeat test a few days later should show falling levels of HCG.

A positive result from either a urine test or a blood test is almost always correct. On the other hand, negative results do sometimes occur even though you are pregnant. This is usually because the test was performed too soon or the urine was too dilute. Most home kits contain two tests so you can repeat the procedure a week later. If you think you have conceived but the tests are giving a negative result, consult your doctor and in the meantime carry on with a healthy diet and lifestyle.

Internal examination Increased blood flow early in pregnancy soon causes the uterus to expand and the colour of the vagina and cervix to deepen. These signs of pregnancy can sometimes be detected by a doctor as early as six to eight weeks from the time of your last period but a blood or urine test will usually confirm a pregnancy before this time.

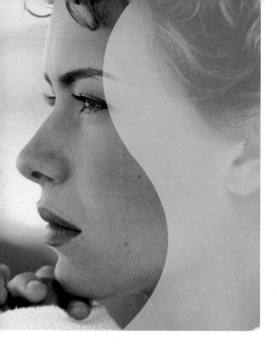

Learning Fertility Awareness

To become aware of your fertile and infertile times, you need to understand the signals your body sends out. Once you have learned fertility awareness, it can reassure you that your cycles are normal and help you pinpoint your most fertile times, increasing your chance of conception. These signals may even tell you if you're pregnant. You can also use fertility awareness to help you avoid pregnancy until you are ready to conceive.

What are your fertility signals?

During your menstrual cycle, your hormones bring about dozens of changes in your body, from the obvious bleeding during a period to changes in the water content of your saliva. The two main changes that you can learn to observe in order to monitor your own fertility are in your cervical mucus and your basal body temperature (BBT). You can also learn to recognise changes in your cervix, breasts and overall mood, giving you extra clues about your fertility from day to day.

Cervical mucus

The cervix is more than just the entrance to the uterus; it has unique features that make it the gateway to your fertility. With a finger, you can feel the lower part of your cervix, near the top of your vagina. It is usually described as being similar to the end of your nose, but is slightly softer and rounder. There is a single dimple in the middle – a small hole called the external cervical os – which is closed during most of the menstrual cycle, but begins to open as ovulation approaches. The cervical os is the entrance to the cervical canal, a passage that is about three centimetres long and lined with mucus-secreting glands. The top of the cervical canal narrows into the internal cervical os which then widens into the cavity of the uterus.

The slight discharge you might notice emerging from your vagina on certain days of your menstrual cycle is secreted by your cervix and vaginal walls. The type of mucus secreted by your cervix depends on the balance of oestrogen and progesterone in your body at that time. Just before ovulation, when oestrogen levels are high, it secretes profuse clear, watery and stretchy mucus. This is the most fertile form of mucus. After ovulation,

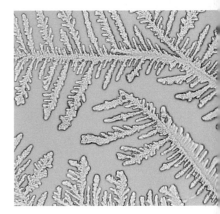

when progesterone levels rise, the mucus becomes thicker and then disappears.

Changes throughout the menstrual cycle Cervical mucus varies constantly during your cycle. After a period, there are usually a few days of vaginal dryness when you notice very little discharge, unless you become sexually aroused or have intercourse. During the first half of your cycle, as soon as oestrogen levels begin to rise, the cervix secretes small amounts of potentially fertile mucus. In a 28-day cycle, cervical mucus usually begins to appear in the second week, around eight to ten days after the start of your period. In longer fertile cycles the cervical mucus appears later. About this time, you may begin to notice a more slippery feel around your vulva or find the occasional blob of sticky mucus on your underwear.

Fertile mucus has an organised crystalline structure that aids the journey of sperm. This can be seen as a ferning pattern when the mucus is viewed under a microscope.

As ovulation approaches, your vagina and vulva will probably feel more lubricated or even wet. The mucus discharged from your vagina increases in quantity and becomes clearer and stretchy until it is like egg white. This type of mucus is called fertile mucus. It provides a nurturing alkaline medium for sperm in the otherwise acid environment of the vagina, and encourages their speedy passage up to the waiting ovum in one of the Fallopian tubes.

The last day that you secrete fertile mucus is known as peak day. You are most fertile during the two or three days that you notice this clear, stretchy mucus leading up to, and including, peak day. After peak day a little opaque-looking mucus may appear for a day or so and the clear, stretchy appearance is lost as the oestrogen levels fall. After you have ovulated you will quickly become drier again around the vulva. This is due to rising levels of progesterone secreted by the ovaries after ovulation. Progesterone causes the mucus at the lower end of the cervix to thicken and form an impenetrable plug, which may help to increase the chance of conception by keeping a reservoir of sperm in the cervical canal after ovulation. Because sperm have a life span of up to five days, this plug allows the maximum time for a sperm to fertilise the waiting ovum successfully. Evidence suggests that fertile mucus is secreted in the upper part of the cervix, while the sticky plug-forming mucus is produced only at the entrance to the cervix, so that the sperm are kept bathed in a pool of fertile mucus.

Factors affecting cervical mucus As you learn to recognise and observe your cervical mucus, it's important to bear in mind that some

How to read your cervical mucus

It takes only a few minutes each day to observe your cervical mucus. Try noticing the sensation around your vulva as you walk about. Is there a feeling of dryness or do the lips of your vagina slip easily as you walk? You can also observe your cervical mucus each time you go to the toilet. Is any mucus on your underwear or on the toilet paper when you wipe yourself? Examine its colour and texture: is it clear, cloudy, stretchy or sticky? See if it stretches between your fingers: fertile mucus is extremely lubricative and may stretch between 7 and 11 cm (3 or 4 in)! If you can't feel any mucus at the vulva try feeling your cervix gently with your fingertip as you should be able to feel mucus there. It's easier to detect these sensations if you wear loose clothing and cotton underwear.

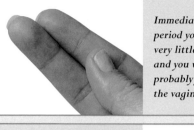

Immediately after your period you will produce very little cervical mucus, and you will most probably feel dry around the vagina.

A few more days into your cycle and you will begin to feel more slippery around your vagina and may notice some sticky or creamy mucus.

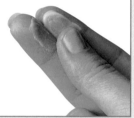

As ovulation nears, your mucus increases in quantity and becomes clear and stretchy. This is a sign of your fertility.

factors can mask its appearance. For example, the day after intercourse you may notice some white or clear discharge. This is liquefied semen, which can easily be confused with cervical mucus. Initially, semen clots, but an hour or so after intercourse it liquefies under the influence of enzymes. Liquefied semen usually disappears within 24 hours of intercourse. Many fertility awareness teachers will advise you to have intercourse only on alternate days before mid-cycle, so that you can identify cervical mucus on the other day. If you are sexually aroused you may get profuse vaginal lubrication, which could be confused with fertile mucus. Try the glass of water test: vaginal secretions on your fingers will dissolve in water but cervical mucus stays in a blob.

If you wear tight clothing your vaginal secretions may be absorbed very quickly, while synthetic materials may make you feel sweaty and damp all the time. Try not to use over-absorbent tampons towards the end of your period as these will dry your vagina. If your period lasts for more

DRUGS THAT CAN AFFECT YOUR CERVICAL MUCUS

Some medications can affect the amount and quality of your cervical mucus, making it more difficult to interpret your fertility signals. If you do need to take any medicines during the preconception period, it's best to check the ingredients listed on the packaging with your doctor or pharmacist.

DRUG	USED TO TREAT	TYPE OF EFFECT
Antidepressants and tranquillizers	Depression, anxiety and sleeping disorders.	May decrease and/or thicken cervical mucus.
Antihistamines	Coughs, colds and hay fever.	
Atropine and dicyclomine	Bowel spasm. Also used as premedication.	
Progestagens	PMS. Also found in contraceptive pills.	
Tamoxifen	Breast cancer and some other breast disorders.	
Cytotoxic drugs	Cancer. Used in chemotherapy.	
Clomiphene	Infertility.	
Danazol	Endometriosis and some breast disorders.	
Cimetidine	Stomach ulcers.	
Acetylcysteine and some other drugs used to clear the lungs	Cystic fibrosis and asthma.	May decrease and/or thin cervical mucus.
Ampicillin (an antibiotic)	Cystitis (bladder inflammation).	
Oestrogens	Menopause. Also found in contraceptive pills.	
Guaifenesin and potassium iodide	Coughs.	
Cholinergic drugs	Urinary retention.	

than a week you may well start secreting cervical mucus towards the end of it. When your menstrual bleeding has stopped, avoid using panty-liners as these can also dry your vulva, making it difficult to detect the early cervical mucus signs.

Many drugs can affect the body's secretions and cervical mucus is no exception. The effects of drugs on cervical mucus vary from one woman to another. In very rare cases a drug can lead to temporary infertility because of its effect on mucus alone (progestagens, for example). Some drugs do affect ovulation, however, and the change in oestrogen levels will have a direct effect on cervical mucus production. Any hormonal contra-

Note	Code	Day
	p	1
	p	2
	p	3
		4
	p	5
	d	6
probably semen	s	7
	d	8
	d	9
A few blobs	s	10
A few blobs	s	11
clear mucus	s	12
stretchy	f	13
wet, stretchy	f	14
clear, stretchy	f	15
dry	d	16
	d	17
	d	18
	d	19
	d	20
probably semen	s	21
	d	22
	d	23
	d	24
	d	25
	d	26
	d	27
see new chart	d	28
		29
		30
		31
		32
		33
		34
		35

Get into the habit of recording the kind of vaginal secretions you notice each day. The chart shown here uses the following abbreviations: p=period; d=dry; s=sticky; f=fertile.

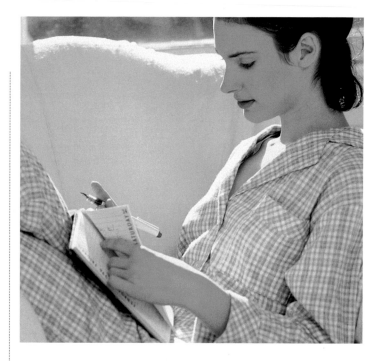

ceptives you take will affect your fertility signals and you will need to stop taking them completely before using fertility awareness for conception or contraception (see also chapter 5). When you are preparing for pregnancy you should always take advice from your doctor or pharmacist before taking a course of medication. For a rundown on drugs that can affect mucus see the chart on page 39.

Recording your cervical mucus As a help in familiarising yourself with your mucus patterns, you should make a mental note throughout the day and record your overall impression on a fertility chart in the evening. Fertility charts are available from fertility awareness teachers. As with your menstrual cycle, fertility charts always count the first day of your period as day one.

When you start charting your vaginal secretions, write down as much detail as possible. Do this until you develop your own consistent code for describing mucus, for example d for dry, s for sticky, p for period, f for fertile, etcetera. Be sure to record when you have sexual intercourse and whether a condom was used – these may affect the amount of discharge you notice the next day. You may also like to note any other signs, such as breast or mood changes, to give you a better idea of how your body changes during your menstrual cycle.

Cervical position and shape

If you find it difficult to notice any mucus secretions try feeling your cervix itself. As well as feeling your mucus you can feel the position of your cervix and the size of the os. As ovulation approaches, your cervix softens and may feel slippery with mucus. The cervical os opens to about the size of your little fingertip. Around this time you may find your cervix easier to feel as it becomes central in the vagina. Early in the menstrual cycle and after ovulation your cervix feels drier and firmer, and the cervical os is closed. Although the cervix may be slightly lower during the infertile phase, it may also be tilted backward and therefore difficult to reach.

To examine your cervix choose a position that you find comfortable. Some women find standing up best, either squatting slightly or with one foot up on a low stool or the edge of the bed. Using the same position each time will help in detecting subtle changes in the consistency, position and shape of your cervix throughout your cycle. Wash your hands and keep your fingernails short and clean. Insert your index finger or index and middle finger, and feel gently at the top of the vagina. Record your findings on your fertility chart.

It will take several months of feeling and recording your cervix to be able to learn your personal patterns of change. After childbirth your cervical os may feel larger and more ragged, so it will take a month or two to recognise the new patterns of change.

Pelvic floor exercises

Learning to use your pelvic floor muscles – the muscles supporting your vagina, bladder and rectum – will help you to detect changes in your vaginal secretions. When cervical mucus is at its most fertile, you will notice a slippery feel between your legs as you use these muscles. At other (less fertile) times, this area feels more dry and your labia separate less easily.

To exercise your pelvic floor muscles, tighten them as if you were desperately needing to use the toilet but had to wait. Hold this for a few seconds then relax and repeat.

Try getting into the habit of contracting and relaxing your pelvic floor muscles a few times every hour or so. Pelvic floor exercises can be done anytime and anywhere – while you wash the dishes, queue at the supermarket, or even talk to a friend on the telephone!

It's important to get good control of your pelvic floor muscles as they will help you strengthen and improve control of your bladder after pregnancy and childbirth. These muscles also can be used to heighten pleasure for both you and your partner during lovemaking.

The position of your cervix and the size of its os (the entrance to the uterus) change throughout your menstrual cycle and is another sign to help you detect your fertile and infertile times.

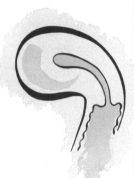

When you are fertile, your cervix is positioned high up, central in the vagina, and the os is wet and open.

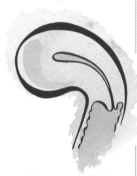

When you are infertile, your cervix is tilted back, may be lower in the vagina, and the os is drier and closed.

Basal body temperature (BBT)

The normal human body temperature averages at about 37°C (98.6°F) but varies during the day, especially in response to exercise. A woman's body temperature not only fluctuates throughout the day, it also responds to hormonal changes throughout the month, thereby giving you valuable information about your fertility cycle. In men and women the body's resting or lowest temperature is called the basal body temperature (BBT).

Changes in BBT In an average 28-day menstrual cycle, with ovulation typically occurring around day 14, the BBT shows two phases. In the first phase, during the menstrual period and through to ovulation, the BBT is at its lowest level. Soon after ovulation, however, the BBT rises at least 0.2°C (approximately 0.4°F) and stays raised until menstruation starts; this is the second or post-ovulatory phase. The rise in temperature is due to the hormone progesterone, which is secreted by the corpus luteum after the ovum has been released, and is a sign that ovulation has already occurred.

Factors affecting BBT As the post-ovulatory rise in BBT is quite small, disturbances in temperature can be confusing. The following are a few of the more common factors that could give a variation in your BBT.

Your body reaches its BBT after you have been asleep for four hours or more, so if you work night shifts or take naps you should take your BBT after your main sleep of the day. If you often get disturbed in the night or early morning, but usually manage to go back to sleep for another couple of hours, remember to record your BBT after your longest sleep. Take your temperature before you get out of bed or have a hot or cold drink because your temperature can change quite quickly.

If you have been drinking alcohol during the evening, your BBT may be high the next morning so don't confuse this with your mid-cycle rise, which should stay raised until your period. Although a hot toddy at night can help you get to sleep, alcohol will actually disturb your sleep so that you sleep less deeply and may cause you to wake up a few hours later. And if you've been up late the night before your BBT may be raised the next morning, which makes for a confusing temperature reading the next day!

Stress, anxiety, illness and infection also can raise your BBT temporarily, as will some drugs that are used to treat menstrual disorders, such as progestagens. Air travel and the resulting jet lag can affect your 24-hour temperature cycle, so bear this in mind when you interpret your overall pattern. If you have repeated, unexplained spikes of high temperature, check that you are shaking down the mercury in your thermometer properly each morning. If you have a sudden dip in temperature it is more likely to be a recording error, so make sure that you are leaving the thermometer in for the required amount of time. An underactive thyroid gland will cause you to have a lower BBT but the effect of this will be to lower every temperature reading rather than to give a sudden dip.

Recording and interpreting your BBT After you have taken your BBT each morning, record it accurately on a chart like the one on page 46. Remember to note any change in health or routine, such as a cold or a party, which may account for an unusual reading. A clear, sustained temperature rise is a good sign that ovulation has occurred.

To help you spot the temperature shift that indicates ovulation, you'll need to draw what is known as a cover line. To do this, identify a row of six lower temperatures on the days after your period has started, then draw a line just above them. This is the cover line over which the post-ovulatory temperature rise will be measured. You can mark this line during the second week of your menstrual cycle if it is usually 28 days long. In cycles that are longer than 28 days, the cover line can be extended over the third week. This rise should be at least $0.2°C$ or $0.4°F$ and will be sustained for the rest of your cycle, until around the first day of your next cycle. When you have recorded three consecutive raised temperatures

How to take your BBT

So that you can take your BBT accurately, you will need to purchase a special glass fertility thermometer which has each degree marked in tenths. You can also use an unbreakable electronic digital thermometer. This is easier to use than a glass thermometer because it makes a beeping sound when a stable temperature is reached. It also stores the information until you are ready to read or record it. If you are using a glass fertility thermometer remember to shake it down well first.

You can record your temperature from your mouth, vagina or rectum but be consistent: your BBT will be slightly different depending on which route you choose. If you use a glass thermometer leave it in place for five minutes before reading the temperature. If the mercury falls between two numbers record the lowest temperature every time. A digital thermometer will need about a minute to "beep" with a temperature reading.

Use a digital thermometer or a glass one specifically designed to take your BBT.

above the cover line, ovulation has probably occurred. However, always check your temperature chart against your cervical mucus chart as mucus changes are the most reliable signs of fertility.

In a fertile cycle, your temperature may start to drop just before your period starts. If you have had sexual intercourse and your ovum has been successfully fertilised, your temperature stays raised. A chart showing a raised temperature for more than 20 days after ovulation may be the first positive sign of your pregnancy.

Other fertility signals

Although cervical mucus is the body's most important signal of fertility, you can learn to recognise other changes in your body that give extra clues to your pattern of fertility.

Sometimes a woman may feel a sharp pain or dull ache low down and to one side of her abdomen when she ovulates. The medical term for this mid-cycle pain is Mittelschmerz, which is German for "middle pain." It may be a momentary twinge or can last for 24 hours and be quite uncomfortable. Studies using ultrasound scans to see what happens when a woman ovulates show that this symptom does not always coincide precisely with ovulation and can be felt just before or after the ovum is released.

A tiny loss of blood sometimes occurs around the time of ovulation, but if you notice this you should see your doctor to check that your cervix is healthy before putting the bleeding down to ovulation. You may also notice that your libido increases around the time of ovulation and decreases again in the infertile days leading up to your period.

You may notice that before your period your breasts become more tender, slightly larger and feel denser or even lumpy. This is due to the progesterone circulating in your body after ovulation. Many women also

If you have been travelling, drinking a lot of alcohol, or have had a late night, note this on your chart as it could raise your temperature. Drawing a cover line will help identify your post-ovulatory temperature rise.

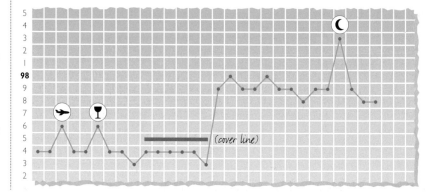

Some reassuring signs of fertility

Amanda came off the pill when she was 25 years old because she and her husband, Joe, were hoping to start a family in the near future. However, Amanda became worried that she might have an infection because she began to notice a vaginal discharge, especially in the week after her period, and sometimes had abdominal pain.

"I was quite concerned and decided to see my doctor. She explained to me that the discharge I had been noticing was cervical mucus, a completely normal sign of my fertility. She mentioned other fertility signs and I recognised the "Mittelschmerz" as being the abdominal pain I sometimes felt. I was very relieved to hear

all this, but I also couldn't believe how little I knew about my own body! My doctor said that being on the pill since I was 16 years old had disguised these signs and she suggested I make a note of them in my diary as a way to help me predict when I was most likely to be fertile.

After a couple of months of charting my mucus and other symptoms, I became very familiar with them. So much so that after one particularly romantic evening when I thought I was at my most fertile, I told Joe that tonight could be the night. Needless to say, he was most impressed when my pregnancy test turned pink four weeks later!"

experience premenstrual changes in mood but these may diminish as you begin to improve your health for pregnancy.

Professor Erik Odeblad of the University of Umea in Sweden has researched widely into fertility awareness and has noticed that some women can detect a small lymph node in their groin that swells when they ovulate. You can test yourself for this lymph node by feeling in your groin during the days when your fertile mucus appears: you may notice a pea-like swelling on one side. Remember, however, that lymph nodes or glands may also swell in this region for many other reasons, for instance, if you have a vaginal infection or flu.

Using fertility awareness to conceive

Now that you have learned about fertility awareness you can use this knowledge to conceive. The most important sign to look for is the slippery, clear and stretchy mucus. If you have intercourse on any of the days that you secrete this mucus you could conceive. However, the most fertile day is usually when the mucus is at its clearest and stretchiest, although not always at its most profuse. If you examine your cervix as well, you will be able to feel as it softens and opens up during your fertile phase.

The rise in your BBT will confirm that your mucus was fertile. Because the temperature rise is caused by progesterone secreted by the corpus luteum after ovulation, it occurs too late to be used as a fertility signal. This BBT rise is usually 12 to 24 hours after ovulation, by which time the ovum has deteriorated and cannot be fertilised. However, if you seem to be having problems getting pregnant, your temperature charts will help you identify possible causes, such as early or late ovulation, lack of ovulation altogether, or even very early miscarriage. Remember, every woman is different and you will need to learn your own unique set of monthly fertility signals.

To optimise your chances of conceiving you should make love when you notice a wet feeling or the slippery, clear mucus. You may not have

Keeping a sympto-thermal chart like the one below will help you become familiar with your body's fertility signals.

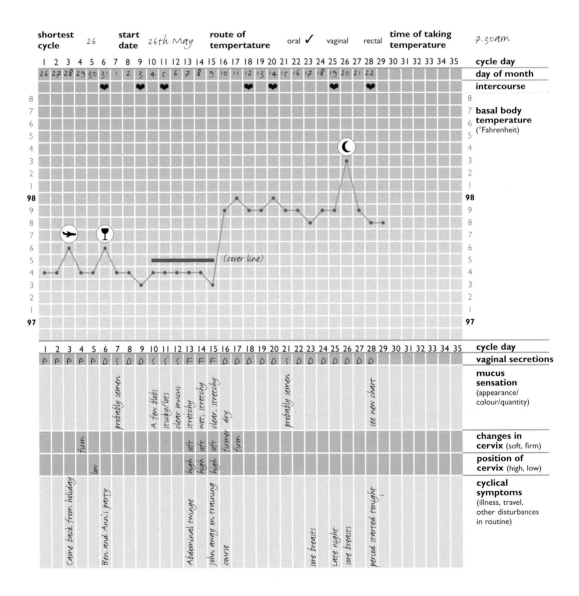

ovulated yet, but fertile mucus is so well designed that it will transport sperm towards the site of fertilisation and nurture them for up to five days, until an ovum is released. Try to have intercourse on the most fertile day (peak day). This is usually the last day you notice fertile mucus and it should soon be followed by the temperature rise which confirms ovulation. Intercourse on one of the five days leading up to the temperature rise is most likely to result in pregnancy.

As fertile mucus helps to nurture and transport sperm, you don't need to have intercourse every day. In fact, having inter- course on alternate days once your cervical mucus appears should not only be sufficient, it may actually help to ensure a higher concentration of sperm in the semen than more fre- quent intercourse. If you don't conceive immediately, don't worry. On average, only one in four fertile couples will con- ceive in a given month, despite having had intercourse at the "right" time.

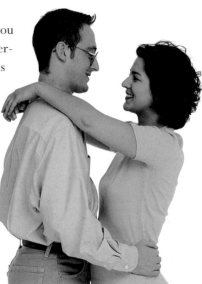

Charting your fertility signs can be a team effort. Involving your partner in this way can make the baby- making experience all the more exciting and intimate.

The symptothermal method of fertility awareness
This method of fertility awareness draws together all the information from the body's fertility signals to help you judge if you are likely to be fertile on a particular day of your cycle. Because it monitors so many physical and emotional changes in each menstrual cycle, it is the most reliable method of fertility awareness. It's important to remember that every woman's fertility signals may vary in timing and nature from the average pattern described in this chapter. A fertility awareness teacher will help you learn to recognise and chart your own, individual fertility signals.

The Billings method of fertility awareness
Since the mid 1960s, the Billings or ovulation method of fertility aware- ness, developed by Drs John and Evelyn Billings, has been taught worldwide. This method relies on a woman recording her daily cervical mucus on a chart, then being taught to recognise her basic infertile pattern of dryness and the arrival of her fertile cervical mucus. Because the Billings method was designed to be completely natural, it doesn't rely on tempera- ture changes as a fertility sign as this would involve the use of a thermometer. This is an advantage in poorer countries where buying and maintaining a thermometer would be impractical, but it means that the Billings method lacks the extra information that temperature readings add to the symptothermal method of fertility awareness.

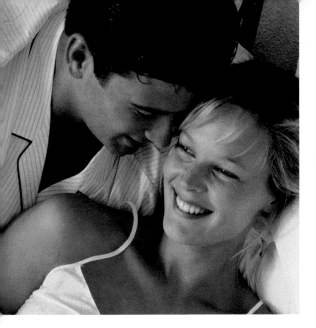

High-tech aids

There are several devices that use the body's natural fertility signals and combine them with modern technology to help you predict your most fertile time. Although these give an accurate result when performed at the right time, they can be expensive and difficult to use if you have an irregular cycle.

Fertility awareness can also be used to avoid pregnancy, yet involves no drugs or devices that might have side effects or interrupt love making.

Ovulation predictor kits These tests use a simple urine test, which detects the surge of luteinising hormone (LH) that triggers ovulation, to help you discover your most fertile time. They are usually very accurate if the urine tests are performed at the right time, but you still need to keep a record of your periods to be able to calculate approximately when you should test for the LH surge.

A typical kit contains five urine-testing sticks which need to be used on consecutive days around the time of ovulation. If you have a regular cycle, you can start testing about 17 days before you expect a period, but if your cycle is at all irregular you could easily miss the five-day fertility window. In this case, you could either buy several kits and test your urine for a much longer time, or you could simply learn to read your cervical mucus, perhaps using a test kit to confirm ovulation.

Computerised fertility predictor This small monitor stores data from your previous menstrual cycles and your daily BBT to predict the days you are fertile. It can be used to indicate infertile times and if your BBT is persistently raised, as in the case of pregnancy. However, it gives a false sense of accuracy because the information it provides is based on previous cycles until your BBT rises, which signals the start of your infertile phase.

Fertility awareness in special situations

Sometimes there are special situations when fertility awareness may help you become aware of your changing fertility, despite having irregular cycles. By learning to recognise your cervical mucus and BBT changes you can learn to predict when you might be fertile during times of low fertility, for instance, whilst breast-feeding, after weight loss, or in the period leading up to the menopause. In these situations intimate knowledge of your body can give you a better picture of your overall fertility pattern than high-tech devices.

After weight loss or stress-related amenorrhoea

If you have been missing periods (amenorrhoea) due to stress or extreme weight loss you may find it reassuring to use a symptothermal chart to monitor your returning fertility. Lack of periods under these circumstances is due to the hypothalamus failing to stimulate ovulation. The first sign of recovery will be some patches of cervical mucus, which indicates that the ovaries are beginning to secrete more oestrogen again. Cervical mucus may come and go for several weeks depending on how fast you are recovering, but will eventually be followed by ovulation and a period.

After a pregnancy ending in miscarriage or termination

Your fertility may return within a week or so of a termination, although this may be longer after a spontaneous miscarriage. To begin with you may find your fertility signs a little confusing. Cervical mucus appears in some women as soon as the initial bleeding has stopped, while others notice a pattern of dryness for a while. Patches of cervical mucus may appear, but without the subsequent temperature rise that would indicate ovulation had occurred. These false alarms are due to rising oestrogen levels, but without ovulation having taken place; they should soon disappear when the menstrual cycle is reestablished. However, if you want to use fertility awareness for contraception, you should regard any cervical mucus as a signal of fertility until it has passed and three dry days have followed. If you are hoping to conceive again soon after losing a pregnancy, first please read Chapter 4: Before You Start. Giving adequate time between pregnancies may be vital to having a healthy baby.

With increasing age

After the age of about 35, most women start to become less fertile and may not ovulate every month, even though they still menstruate regularly. A slight shortening of the "monthly" menstrual cycle is common with age. If you are hoping to conceive and age is not on your side, you can use fertility charts to increase your chances of conceiving by determining your most fertile time and having sexual intercourse at that time. Chapter 4 offers more detail on the effects of age on fertility and pregnancy.

During treatment for cervical problems

If the cervix is damaged or becomes infected, your fertility may be affected (see also page 155). If you have received treatment for an abnormal cervical smear or cervical cancer, such as a loop excision (when the affected tissue is removed from the tip of the cervix), or a cone biopsy (when the

Ovulation predictor kits test your urine for levels of LH (luteinising hormone), the chemical that triggers ovulation.

Fertility awareness after childbirth

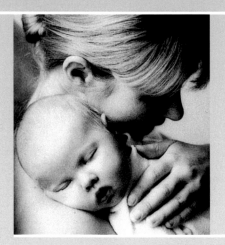

Fertility takes some time to return after pregnancy and if you breast-feed, your menstrual cycle may rest for many months. This is because the hormone prolactin is released by the pituitary gland, which inhibits the ovaries' production of oestrogen. As a result, the hypothalamus and pituitary do not send out the surge of LH that stimulates ovulation.

If you breast-feed

In the early weeks of breast-feeding, you will begin to notice a constant pattern to your vaginal secretions, rather than the changing one in your usual fertile cycle. The secretions will probably be slightly more moist than the dry days you used to notice after ovulation, but won't contain cervical mucus and may be slightly cloudy. While you are fully breast-feeding (that is, your baby has no extra juice or solid foods and is probably nursing every two to four hours) this pattern tends to be the same day after day. Any change should inform you that your fertility may be returning.

If you start recording your BBT a few weeks after your baby's birth, it will typically show wide swings of up to 0.4°C (1°F) during breast-feeding, which may be partly due to sleep disturbance. Your BBT may start to level off when your first ovulation approaches and you should interpret this and the appearance of any mucus as a sign that you may be fertile.

If you would like to learn fertility awareness while breast-feeding, seek the help of a trained teacher. Your charts should include details of your baby's health and feeding patterns to help you recognise how these can affect your fertility signals. Most natural family planning teachers will have special charts for breast-feeding mothers.

If you don't breast-feed

You may become fertile within a month of so of your baby's birth, although this is unusual: two months is more common. Most mothers who don't breast-feed will have normal periods again by about 12 weeks (and some much earlier), although the first bleed may come before the first ovulation and is not a true period. Keeping a symptothermal chart will enable you to see your fertility return. It's possible to start ovulating as early as 21 to 28 days after delivery, so if you don't breast-feed and don't want another baby straight away, start using contraception two or three weeks after having your baby.

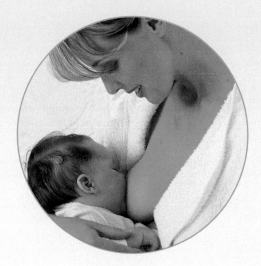

damage is more extensive and a cone-shaped piece of tissue is removed from the cervix) you may notice a change in your cervical mucus depending on how extensive the treatment was. Usually the treatment for an abnormal smear of cervical cancer will only remove the surface of the cervix near the external os, the area known as the transformation zone. The upper part of the cervical canal remains undamaged so it can still produce cervical mucus. Studies of women trying to conceive after loop excision biopsy of the transformation zone (LETZ) have been encouraging and most women can go on to have a normal pregnancy if they are otherwise healthy.

If you suffer from an unusual or continuous discharge after treatment and have found it difficult to recognise the sort of fertile mucus pattern described in this chapter, you should have a medical check-up to make sure that you are not suffering from a cervical infection. Although harmless, cervical erosion may also cause an abnormal vaginal discharge, making fertility awareness difficult. These cervical problems should be checked by your doctor and, if necessary, treated before you embark on a pregnancy.

?

DID YOU KNOW?

The first scientific trials of natural family planning methods were not published until the 1970s, but at least three Kenyan tribes (the Taita, the Kamba and the Luo), as well as an Australian Aboriginal tribe (the Niranji), are known to have taught their young women for many generations the cervical mucus signs to detect fertility.

Three steps to conception

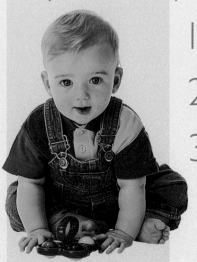

It may take a few cycles for you to become familiar with your body's natural fertility signs, but once you do, you will have a much better idea of when the right time to conceive will be. Just remember that there are three golden rules to using fertility awareness in order to get pregnant. These are to have intercourse on the days when your:

1 Cervical mucus is fertile (clear and stretchy).

2 Basal body temperature has not yet risen.

3 Cervix is high, soft, open and central in the vagina.

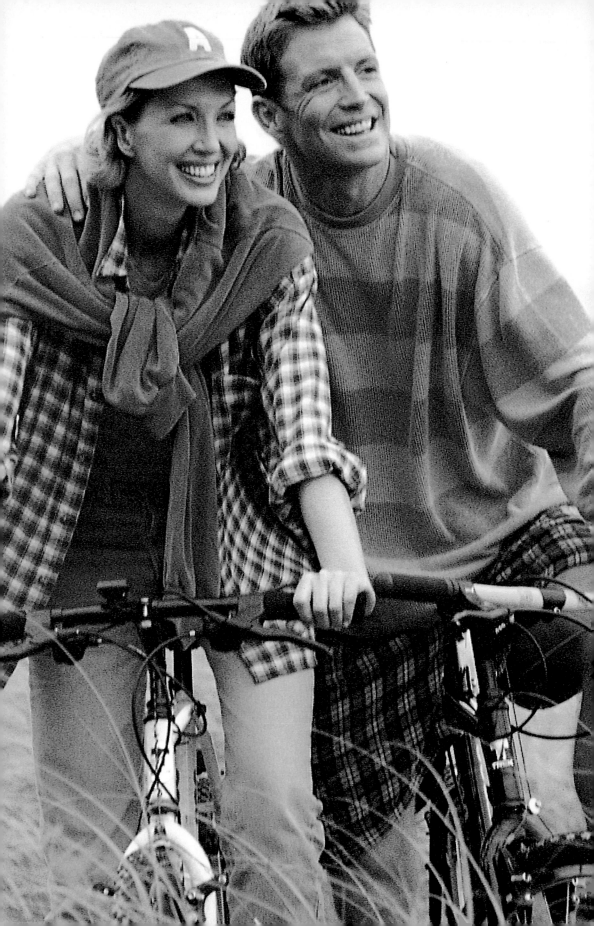

PART II

GETTING READY
TO CONCEIVE

*Starting a family is an exciting decision that will affect many
aspects of your life. But far from the outcome of your
pregnancy being a matter of fate, there are many proactive
things you can do to work with your body's natural
ability to conceive and carry a baby successfully.
The following chapters will show how you and your
partner can improve your health and lifestyle
during the crucial preconception period.*

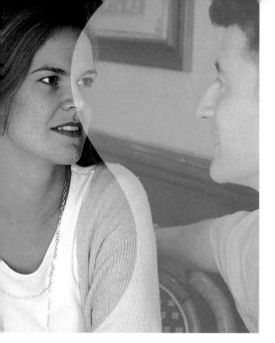

Before You Start

Once you have made the exciting decision to go ahead and have a family, you and your partner will probably want to get started right away. But before you do, it's important to take some time to consider certain factors. As well as good physical health and emotional well-being, the space you leave between one pregnancy and the next (even if the pregnancy hasn't gone to full term), and your age and that of your partner can have an important impact on conception, your health during pregnancy, and your baby's health after birth.

Reviewing your health

Your health and that of your partner play a vital role in your ability to conceive and sustain a pregnancy successfully. What's more, because pregnancy is very physically demanding, the healthier you are at the outset, the better equipped your body will be to carry and nourish your baby throughout pregnancy.

The following chapters in this part of the book will guide you to developing a healthier lifestyle and show you how, by taking control of specific areas in your life, you can boost your fertility and improve your chances of getting pregnant. For instance, while you improve your health for conception you will need to choose a suitable form of contraception and chapter 5 outlines your choices. From the moment your baby is conceived your body will need a good supply of nutrients and chapter 6 tells you which foods to choose from in order to give your baby the best start in life. Improving your physical fitness and managing emotional factors such as stress, anxiety and depression may sound daunting, but it can be done and go a long way in helping you to enjoy your pregnancy. This is discussed in chapter 7. If you are a smoker, chapter 8 details how important it is to quit, as well as avoiding other harmful habits. Even if you don't smoke, you might need to reduce your exposure to other toxins and environmental hazards, and this is discussed in chapter 9. Finally, if you or your partner has a long-term health problem you will most certainly benefit from the advice in chapter 10 concerning this and other medical conditions which may affect your fertility or pregnancy.

You may also find it helpful if you and your partner visit your local doctor or family planning clinic for a general health check-up during this preconception period. For more information on what to be tested for at your preconception check-up, turn to page 169.

You may already have strong views on the ideal age gap between children in a family: some parents want to have children close enough to be play-mates, while others shudder at the thought of simultaneous nappy and potty training, or worry about jealousy between siblings. Whatever your ideas regarding the ideal family, it's important to know that your chance of a healthy pregnancy and the health of your children may be affected by the gap you leave between one pregnancy and the next.

Pregnancy makes high demands on your body, even in the early weeks after conception. This means that the time you give your body to recover after having a baby (or suffering a miscarriage) can have an important impact on your health during your next pregnancy. If you become preg-nant too soon after your last pregnancy, you run an increased risk of having a miscarriage and your baby may be at risk of being born underweight. Babies conceived too soon after a previous pregnancy may also be more likely to suffer from birth defects, or not survive around the time of birth.

What is a safe birth interval?

In 1970 the results of a survey of pregnant women in the UK showed that the classic two-year age gap between children was associated with the healthiest outcome for each baby. The results estimated that 13 per cent of babies born with dangerously low birth weights or who died soon after birth could be accounted for by the pregnancy being spaced too closely to another, even when other risks such as smoking during pregnancy were allowed for.

A World Health Organization study published in 1981 showed that women all over the world, including Australia, Hawaii, Pakistan, Egypt and Saudi Arabia, had increased risks to the health of their second or sub-sequent baby when the interval between pregnancies was shorter than a year. In one US survey, out of a million births, the risk of having a baby with low birth weight was three times greater if the baby was conceived only three months after the previous birth, compared to babies conceived two years or more after a previous birth.

The risk of miscarriage also increases if one pregnancy follows another too quickly, and this risk seems greatest in countries where women are poorly nourished, live in sub-standard housing and have little access to health care. For instance, a survey in Pakistan showed that over

Spacing your pregnancies

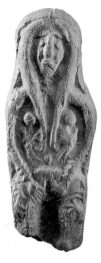

Getting pregnant is no longer a matter of praying to a fertility charm, such as this Ancient Egyptian figurine. Improving your health will increase your chances of conceiving.

60 per cent of pregnancies conceived within a year of the last ended in miscarriage. Another study in Turkey showed 37 per cent of pregnancies conceived less than four months after the last pregnancy were lost. However, close spacing of pregnancies can affect mothers in the affluent West as well.

If you had a problem in a previous pregnancy, such as an ectopic pregnancy, miscarriage or pre-eclampsia, it's natural that you should worry about getting pregnant again. To give yourself the best chance of a healthy pregnancy in the future, you should leave enough time for your body to recover from the previous pregnancy – at least a year between one conception and the next after a full-term pregnancy – and use this time to improve your health. For more information and advice on problems in previous pregnancies, see page 158.

Does your age matter?

More and more couples are choosing to wait longer before beginning their families and often don't start trying for babies until they are well into their 30s. If you are among them, you may be worrying about how long it will take you to conceive or feel concerned about the outcome of a pregnancy

Second time lucky

Jodie and Mark were ready to start a family, but when Jodie's first pregnancy ended in miscarriage after only a few weeks, they were unsure about trying again soon afterward.

"Mark and I had always wanted to become parents, so you can imagine how devastated we were when I started bleeding in my eighth week. We wanted to try for another baby right away, but Mark thought we ought to talk to our doctor first. The doctor was very reassuring and told us that as this was my only miscarriage, the chances of it happening again were small. He did advise us, however, that we should wait for about three months to let my body recover.

He also suggested we look at our diet and lifestyle to see if we could improve it in any way. We had both been busy and not eating proper meals, and Mark admitted that he had been stressed at work and drinking quite a bit. We decided to make a big effort not to eat on the run and spend more time shopping for groceries, cooking and sitting down to a healthy meal in the evenings. On our doctor's advice I started taking folic acid supplements and Mark cut down his alcohol intake to just the occasional drink.

After a few months I was feeling really fit and healthy. I had had two normal periods and we felt confident enough to try again for a baby. A couple of weeks later I discovered I was pregnant!

Mark and I carried on with our healthy diet and lifestyle and, after a problem-free pregnancy, Ben – our pride and joy – was born!"

once you decide to proceed. But even though you may no longer be at the peak of your fertility, you'll be relieved to know that the chances of having a successful pregnancy and birth are very good, provided you and your partner are both fit and healthy.

For "older" mums

There is no doubt that the healthiest time for a woman to embark on a pregnancy is before the age of 35, but there is certainly nothing magical about this age. For a healthy woman who becomes pregnant in her late 30s, the outlook is good. Health risks for both mother and baby during

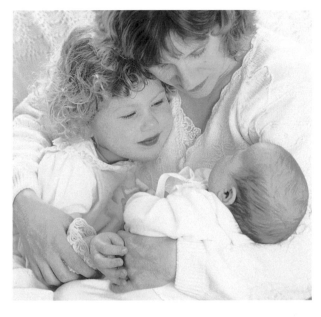

pregnancy do increase with age, but much of this risk is linked to medical problems that increase with age. For example, blood pressure tends to rise with age and may increase the mother's risk of developing pre-eclampsia during pregnancy (see page 159). Some women put on weight with age and because obesity is associated with diabetes, this can be a risk factor for both mother and baby during pregnancy.

Research indicates that it is better to wait at least two years after the birth of one baby before conceiving another. This baby is enjoying the attention of both her mother and sister.

Consequently, if you are healthy, your age alone probably won't increase the risks during your pregnancy very much. Research has shown that with good prenatal care, pregnancy and childbirth can be just as safe for healthy older women and their babies as they are for younger women.

The risk of miscarriage This does increase with age and can be a frequent source of disappointment for older women planning families. However, miscarriage is more common than you might think in women of all ages: around 50 per cent of all fertilised ova do not develop into a pregnancy and many are lost with the next period without ever implanting into the uterus. In women under the age of 35, as many as one in ten pregnancies ends in miscarriage (although some of these occur before women are aware they are pregnant and are noticed only as a late or heavy period). For women over the age of 40, on average, the figure rises to about one in five. But do not let these statistics deter you if you are in the latter part of your fertile years and are hoping to conceive: at least 80 per cent of pregnancies do not end in miscarriage, even in mothers over the age of 40!

What causes miscarriage? At least half of all conceptions lost during pregnancy have chromosomal disorders – so miscarriage seems to be Nature's way of ensuring that the majority of babies born are healthy. This is especially the case in older women, although there is a tendency for perfectly healthy conceptions to be miscarried in older women too.

Age is not the only factor, though: older mothers are more likely to have medical problems, such as diabetes (see page 163), which increase the risk of miscarriage. Again, don't be deterred from trying to conceive: you can take positive action to reduce the risks of miscarriage by following the preconception advice set out in the following chapters. If you are in good health and take good prenatal care, you probably do not have a high risk of miscarriage or stillbirth. Interestingly, the risk of miscarriage for an older, healthy woman if she has already had a healthy baby is lower than the average one in five – even if she embarks on a second or third pregnancy much later in life.

OVULATION AND FERTILITY

For every ten couples in their 20s, eight or nine can expect to conceive within a year of trying. However for women over the age of 40, only four or five out of every ten will conceive. Only one in ten women over the age of 45 can expect to become pregnant within a year of trying. The reason for this last statistic is mainly due to the fact that in the ten years leading up to the menopause, a woman may only ovulate, on average, in eight menstrual cycles each year. The reason why ovulatory cycles are not always fertile is not fully understood, but may be due to the corpus luteum failing to survive the full two weeks needed to establish a pregnancy, or the uterus not being receptive to the released ovum because of low progesterone and oestrogen levels.

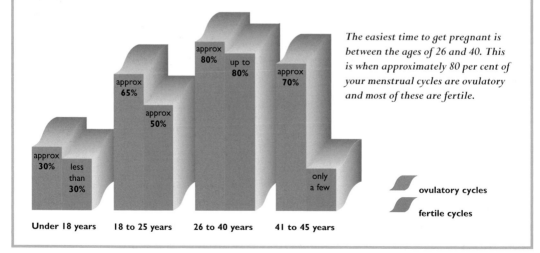

The easiest time to get pregnant is between the ages of 26 and 40. This is when approximately 80 per cent of your menstrual cycles are ovulatory and most of these are fertile.

approx 80%
up to 80%
approx 65%
approx 70%
approx 50%
approx 30%
less than 30%
only a few

ovulatory cycles

fertile cycles

Under 18 years   18 to 25 years   26 to 40 years   41 to 45 years

Will my baby be normal? While a few women seem to sail serenely through preconception and pregnancy, I suspect that almost every woman experiences the fear of this unanswered question at times. That is, until the joyful day she holds her healthy baby in her arms. For older women, this worry can be particularly intense.

Around 1 in 50 babies is born with some birth defect, leaving 98 per cent of all babies born healthy. Most of these defects are not inherited or related to the parents' age. However, older women are more likely to have a pregnancy affected by chromosomal problems, which could result in a miscarriage or the baby being affected by Down's syndrome (see also page 60). The overall risk of having a baby with a birth defect is greatest at the two extremes of the fertile years. This means that mothers under the age of 15 or over 45 have twice the average risk of having a baby with birth defects. Age does not seem to have a significant effect between the ages of 20 and 40.

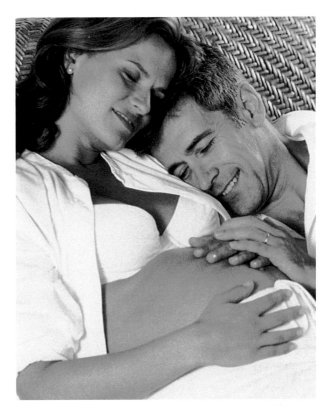

Pregnancy should be a very positive experience irrespective of your age, especially if you and your partner take good care of your health.

Social considerations Whenever you decide to become a parent, you will find that your age brings with it some advantages, as well as challenges. Young mums are often thought to adapt better to the physical demands of parenthood, but mothers of all ages can find pregnancy and the early days of motherhood tiring. Having a positive outlook will help carry you through many of the difficulties of parenting, irrespective of your age.

Young mothers may feel more in touch with the childhood and teenage struggles their children face, but as an older mother you will have maturity on your side. After mixing and working with many different people over the years, you also may be much more tolerant. As an older first-time mum, you may find it hard to adjust to your new role after many years without children. But one of the hallmarks of human nature is our ability to adapt, and you may surprise yourself by how naturally you take to motherhood. You may feel socially alienated, especially at play groups where other mums can seem young enough to be your daughters, but don't let this deter you! As more and more women are choosing to have their babies later in life, you are quite likely to meet many other older mums anywhere from your prenatal classes to outside the school gates.

DOWN'S SYNDROME

This chromosomal disorder can result when there is a failure in the formation of the ovum or sperm, which causes them to carry extra material from chromosome 21. Down's syndrome is also called Trisomy 21 as there can be three, rather than the usual pair of chromosome 21. It can also occur when the chromosomes do not separate properly at the time of fertilisation. Very occasionally, it may be caused when one parent has an abnormal balance of chromosome 21, which does not affect the parent but can be passed on to the children.

Children with Down's syndrome have characteristic facial features and often have a very friendly disposition. They usually have special educational needs, although some can be catered for in normal schools. Some Down's syndrome children suffer from congenital heart defects and other physical handicaps, but it is their learning difficulties that make them unlikely to lead an independent life during adulthood.

MOTHER'S AGE	APPROXIMATE RISK
20 years	1 in 2000 babies
30 years	1 in 900 babies
35 years	1 in 400 babies
40 years	1 in 100 babies
45 years	1 in 30 babies
50 years	1 in 12 babies

About 1 in 800 babies is affected by Down's syndrome. Although the risk does rise with maternal age, most affected babies have younger mothers because more babies are born to mothers under the age of 30. It's difficult to interpret these figures into tangible risks for each mother-to-be personally, but to interpret them more positively, only 1 in 100 babies born to 40-year-old mothers will have Down's syndrome. This means that 99 per cent of babies born to women aged 40 will not have Down's syndrome. Several screening tests (see pages 62–63) are available during pregnancy to help identify women at risk of carrying a baby with Down's syndrome.

Most people with Down's syndrome have 47 chromosomes instead of the normal 46, because they carry an extra chromosome 21.

For "older" dads

Men don't experience a menopause when their fertility comes to an abrupt halt and, as a consequence,
many men remain fertile all their lives. Because of
this they are capable of fathering a child well after
the retirement age for most other occupations!
Semen quality does decline with age but even
though the overall sperm count tends to fall, Nature
leaves a wide safety margin and most men still have
enough sperm to be fertile well into old age.

As well as falling sperm count, the number of
fully motile sperm and the overall volume of semen
decrease slightly with age. Generally, these changes
aren't noticeable until after a man reaches his 50s
and, even then, the effects are not significant until
his mid 60s.

Overall, for healthy, fit men, the effects of age
on fertility are very small and other issues such as
smoking (see chapter 8) and general fitness (see
chapter 7) are much more important in determining
semen quality. Although age is something to take
into consideration when you are planning your
family, factors such as financial considerations and
social implications will probably be much more
important to you.

Age and male sexual behaviour As a man gets
older, not only does his sperm count decrease, his
sexual response may change too. Most men tend to
find that as they age, they take longer to become
sexually aroused and have fewer spontaneous erec-
tions. This is due in part to falling testosterone levels, which decrease at a
rate of one per cent a year from the age of 35. However, because the
normal range of testosterone levels is very wide, some 80-year-old men
can have testosterone levels equal to some 20-year-old men! Generally
speaking, a man at the age of 80 has about half the level of testosterone he
had at the age of 30.

As a man ages, many of his vital organs suffer from decreasing blood
supply. This is particularly the case if stress and a high-fat diet have allowed
atherosclerosis (a furring up or hardening in the arteries) to occur. The

TIME TO TALK

Are you ready for parenthood?

*Starting a family is like setting out on an
exciting adventure across uncharted territo-
ry. Some couples feel daunted by it, while
other couples take the first steps without a
backward glance. There may not be a perfect
time when all your health, social and financial issues are ideal, but you can help to
prepare for parenthood by taking the time to
discuss the following points with your
partner:*

- How will your relationship change
  during pregnancy, the early years of
  parenthood and beyond?
- How will you be able to help your
  children grow up fulfiled and responsible?
- What are your hopes and wishes for
  their education and future?
- What are your views on discipline?
- Who will care for your baby if you
  both plan to keep working?
- Will you be able to manage financially
  if you decide one of you should stop
  working altogether?

Screening tests during pregnancy

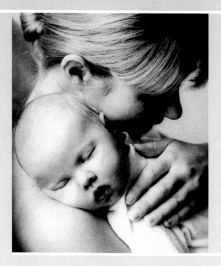

Both you and your baby will be carefully monitored to ensure your pregnancy is progressing well. Part of this prenatal care includes screening tests to help detect some birth defects. These tests do not usually give a diagnosis, but indicate whether further, more accurate tests are necessary. This can be stressful so you need to be fully informed to keep any development in perspective. Make sure you know what each test is for, its accuracy, if there are any risks for you or your baby, and what can be done if the test shows an abnormality.

Ultrasound scans

The most common screening test during pregnancy is the ultrasound scan. This uses high-frequency sound waves to display an image of your unborn baby and placenta on a screen. Ultrasound scans can show your baby's heart beating as early as eight to ten weeks of pregnancy, while later scans can show details of your baby's face and genitals – thus revealing its sex – and some developmental abnormalities, such as spina bifida (where the spinal column does not fuse to protect the spinal cord, often leading to paralysis) and anencephaly (an undeveloped skull and brain).

Ultrasound scanning techniques have come a long way since the first hazy image produced in the late 1960s. Scans are most useful as a way to answer specific questions, such as the age of the baby (scans taken in the first trimester can predict this to within five days), whether he is lying in a breech or head-down position, and if his growth rate is normal.

Alpha feto protein (AFP) test

In recent years obstetricians have developed combinations of blood tests for pregnant women to try to detect mothers at risk of having a baby with Down's syndrome or spina bifida. Most of these tests include measuring the amount of alpha feto protein (AFP) in the blood. Pregnant women carrying babies with spina bifida have higher levels of AFP. If a baby

has Down's syndrome, AFP circulates in low levels. Mothers-to-be who are shown to have a high risk of a Down's syndrome baby are offered more definitive tests, like amniocentesis and chorionic villus sampling. More recently, AFP tests are being replaced by the triple test, which is taken at 16 weeks of pregnancy. In addition to AFP levels, this test measures human chorionic gonadotrophin (HCG) and oestriol levels to help identify mothers at risk of carrying babies with Down's syndrome. However, even with screening some babies with abnormalities will be missed.

The normal levels of these chemicals measured in tests vary according to what week of pregnancy a woman is in, so it's important to remember that, to be reliable, these tests require accurate conception dates. Often, a false alarm is raised because a woman's pregnancy is inaccurately dated. An early ultrasound scan or well-kept fertility charts (see page 47) will help you accurately date your baby's conception.

Amniocentesis

This involves inserting a long, fine needle through a pregnant woman's abdomen to draw out some of the amniotic fluid surrounding her unborn baby. (Amniocentesis is usually performed under ultrasound guidance to determine the position of the baby.) The chromosomes from the cells in this fluid are then studied and chromosomal defects can be determined. The sex of your child can also be detected, which is important if a sex-linked inherited disorder, such as haemophilia, is suspected.

Amniocentesis is usually performed at 16 weeks of pregnancy and carries a 1 per cent risk of miscarriage. In other words, there is a 99 per cent chance that you will not miscarry after the test. The procedure only takes a few minutes, but the results may take a month to come back. This waiting period can be an anxious time for parents-to-be, but the test will usually give a definite answer to whether their child has a specific chromosomal disorder, such as Down's syndrome.

Chorionic villus sampling (CVS)

This also tests for genetic and chromosomal abnormalities, but is usually only undertaken when a specific disorder, such as cystic fibrosis, is suspected. A fine needle is used to draw out some of the tissue (called chorionic villi) growing at the edge of the placenta, which contains the same genetic information as the foetal cells. CVS may be performed vaginally or through the abdomen and is usually carried out around 11 weeks of pregnancy. Although it can be carried out

earlier than amniocentesis, there is a 2 to 5 per cent risk of miscarriage or stillbirth. Put more positively, there is a 95 to 98 per cent chance that CVS will not cause miscarriage or stillbirth.

Screening tests vary around the country and you should discuss with your midwife or GP what tests you are likely to be offered and how accurate they are. Of course, the bottom line with screening tests is what to do if your baby is diagnosed with a disorder? With most major abnormalities, medical science can only offer a termination of the pregnancy. Occasionally new developments in foetal surgery hit the headlines but, at present, very few birth defects or inherited problems can be treated in utero. If you could not accept a termination you may decide that some of these tests are not for you. On the other hand, just knowing ahead of time may help you prepare for the future. This is an issue that every couple needs to decide for themselves.

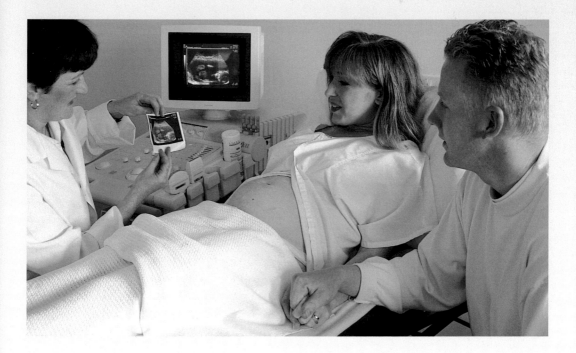

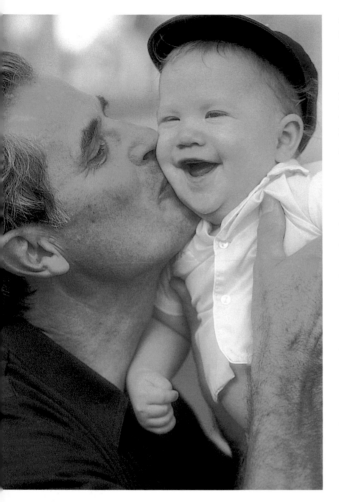

Men don't face the predicament of the biological clock in quite the same way as women and can usually father a healthy child well past the age of 40.

arteries become narrow and the poor blood supply that results reduces the production of testosterone in the testes. So, if you are an older man and you are planning to start a family, make sure you keep physically fit as this will help to improve the blood supply to your testes, and thereby reduce the effects of ageing.

Is paternal age a risk factor for birth defects? On the whole, there is very little link between most birth defects and paternal age, although there are some exceptions. The results of a large study in British Columbia, Canada concluded that out of a sample of nearly 10,000 babies born between 1952 and 1973, older men tended to father more babies with spina bifida, congenital cataracts, some rare limb defects and Down's syndrome. It also showed an increase risk of birth defects in babies born to men under 20 years, although the risks were marginal.

In particular, men over the age of 50 were twice as likely as men aged between 25 and 29 to have a baby with spina bifida. As about 1 in 600 conceptions are affected by spina bifida, this still only gives a risk of perhaps 1 in 300 for fathers over 50 years. The risks of contracting some genetic diseases such as achondroplasia (dwarfism) increase slightly with paternal age and this is thought to be due to copying errors in the chromosomes during sperm production. However, even with increasing age, the risks for most genetic diseases are low. For example, only about 1 in 10,000 babies are born with achondroplasia, and although the risk is increased tenfold in fathers over 50, this still only gives a 1 in 1,000 risk.

It's important to remember that many babies conceived with defective sperm will be lost through miscarriage. So, although the link between paternal age and birth defects is minimal, women with much older partners have an increased risk of miscarriage.

If you are concerned about the effects your age may have on the health of your baby or think there may be an inherited illness running in your family, you may like to consider having genetic counselling. If you or your partner suffer from any long-term health problem (see chapter 10) you may also want to get some advice on whether this is likely to affect your children.

A genetic counsellor is usually a doctor with special training in inherited diseases. Counselling commonly starts with both you and your partner giving as much information as possible about your health and those of your close relatives. In order to do this you will need to find out as much as you can about all the children born on both sides of your family for the last three generations. If you or a close relative suffers from a medical problem, an accurate diagnosis is required and this may involve medical tests. Sometimes there are no surviving children in affected families or it may be an upsetting subject to discuss, particularly for elderly relatives. In this case you'll need to make discreet inquiries from other relatives to find out, for example, if you have an aunt who suffered repeated miscarriages or unexplained infertility.

You may wonder why all couples aren't offered tests to screen for inherited diseases but it is not that simple. Genetic counselling can be a long and involved process of investigation and even though many hundreds of genetic tests can now be performed, each one is very expensive. At present it is practical only to test for gene disorders when there is a very strong chance a conception might be affected.

Genetic counselling

Who should have genetic counselling?

If one of the following statements applies to you or your partner, you could ask for genetic counselling. It's important to remember that there may be no accurate test for the medical condition that is concerning you, and you will probably only be given a risk factor (rather than a definite prediction) that your baby may be affected.

- You have already had a baby with a health problem or birth defect.
- There is a health problem that seems to run in your or your partner's family.

- You or your partner has a brother or sister who has a serious birth defect.
- You or your partner has a serious medical problem or birth defect and you worry that you or he may be a carrier (see box on page 66).
- You consider yourselves to be older parents (for instance, over 40 for a woman and over 50 for a man).
- You have had several miscarriages or a stillbirth.
- You and your partner are first cousins, or otherwise closely related.

INHERITED DISORDERS

Most inherited diseases can be passed on from one generation to the next by a very small fault in one of the thousands of genes on each chromosome. This is called a gene mutation. During meiosis, when the chromosomes divide and new sperm or ovum are formed, some will carry the faulty gene that causes the illness.

Some genetic disorders, such as achondroplasia (dwarfism), will affect every person carrying the faulty gene and are therefore known as dominant genetic disorders. In these cases the faulty gene is present on one of each pair of the affected chromosomes and will be passed on to one in two of the parent's children, who will also be affected by the disorder.

Other genetic disorders, such as cystic fibrosis (see page 168), are known as recessive genetic disorders; children will only be affected if they inherit faulty genes from both parents. Recessive genetic disorders will be passed on to all of the affected parent's children, but unless the child also inherits a defective gene from the other parent he or she will only be a carrier of the disorder. Recessive gene problems are more likely to occur when close relatives, such as cousins, or those from a closely knit ethnic group have a child.

If the faulty recessive gene is on the X chromosome then the disorder is said to be sex linked. Haemophilia is passed on in this way. Usually only boys are affected because they have just one X chromosome. Girls who inherit a faulty X chromosome generally have no symptoms because the normal gene on their second X chromosome will compensate. Affected fathers can only pass this on to their daughters who become carriers, and who in turn will pass it on to half their own sons. Affected fathers' sons cannot inherit the condition.

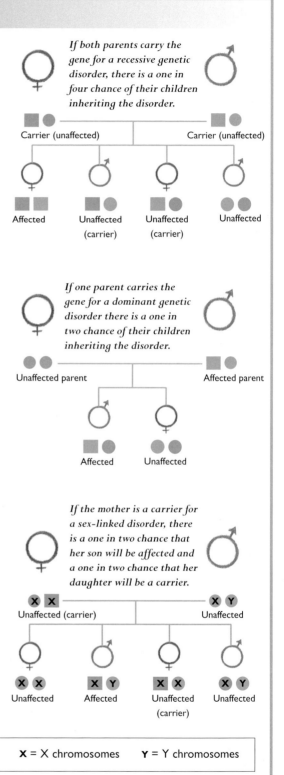

If both parents carry the gene for a recessive genetic disorder, there is a one in four chance of their children inheriting the disorder.

Carrier (unaffected)   Carrier (unaffected)

Affected   Unaffected   Unaffected   Unaffected
              (carrier)   (carrier)

If one parent carries the gene for a dominant genetic disorder there is a one in two chance of their children inheriting the disorder.

Unaffected parent   Affected parent

Affected   Unaffected

If the mother is a carrier for a sex-linked disorder, there is a one in two chance that her son will be affected and a one in two chance that her daughter will be a carrier.

X X   X Y
Unaffected (carrier)   Unaffected

X X   X Y   X X   X Y
Unaffected   Affected   Unaffected   Unaffected
                          (carrier)

■ ■ Defective genes   ● ● Normal genes   **X** = X chromosomes   **Y** = Y chromosomes

When planning a baby, most couples do not give the season of their child's birth much thought. But there are some social and medical advantages to being born at certain times of the year. In the animal kingdom, for instance, most mothers tend to have their babies in the spring when the weather is warm and food supplies are guaranteed.

Is there a right season to be born?

One important reason to time the birth of your baby to a particular month is the correlation between the seasons and the risk of developing allergies, such as hay fever or asthma. Babies who are born to parents with allergic tendencies are at a higher risk of developing allergies, particularly if they are exposed to allergens in the first three to six months of their lives.

For instance, in the UK, babies born between March and September are most likely to develop hay fever. A baby conceived between December and July is least likely to develop hay fever. Asthma is commonly due to an allergy to the house dust mite, which thrives in warm, centrally heated, carpeted and draught-proof houses. This may explain why babies born in the winter are more likely to develop asthma. If you are having a winter baby, you can cut down on his exposure to dust by making sure his room is frequently cleaned, has good ventilation, and contains very little soft furnishings, such as cushions. Washable rugs on a polished floor make a good substitute for carpeting. Research has indicated that breast-fed babies are least likely to develop an allergy, no matter what season they are born.

You may have more personal reasons for wanting to time your baby's birth for a particular month in the year. For example, if you are a teacher, you may want to coincide the birth with school holidays. You may also want to avoid having your child's birthday very close to the beginning of the academic year, as this could make her either very young or very old for her school year. Alternatively, perhaps you'd like to keep your child's birthday away from Christmas or that of another close relative. This, however, is very fine tuning that most parents don't consider, especially as conception rarely happens to order!

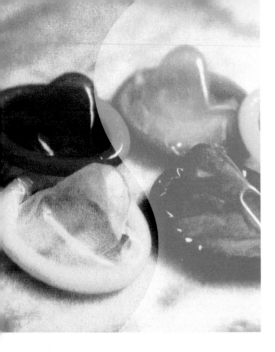

Contraception While You Prepare For Pregnancy

Now that you are thinking of getting pregnant, it may seem natural to throw your pills away and let nature take its course. But before you do, allow plenty of time for any health improvements. While preparing for pregnancy you will want to use a contraceptive that delays conception until you're ready to conceive, but does not affect your fertility.

Are you using the best form of contraception?

An essential part of your preconception care program is deciding whether you need to change to a more suitable contraceptive while you prepare for pregnancy. The method you choose is very much a matter of personal preference but, ideally, should be one that is safe and reliable, has few medical side effects, and is easily reversible once you are ready to conceive.

Hormonal methods

Many women using contraceptive pills, injections, the intrauterine system (IUS) and implants want to know whether they will have difficulty conceiving once they stop using these contraceptives. Although all hormonal contraceptives work by inhibiting the natural fertility cycle, the time it takes for your fertility to normalise after stopping them depends on the particular type you have been using. For example, although the combined oral contraceptive pill (one of the most popular forms of contraception in the UK and US) prevents ovulation, your body can recover quite quickly after coming off it. The same applies to the progestagen-only pill, implants and the intrauterine system, which all work by thickening the cervical mucus to prevent sperm getting through (and preventing ovulation in some women).

Progestagen injections, on the other hand, can cause long delays to your ovulation returning, so it is important that you allow a significant period of time after stopping this method of contraception before intending to conceive. In the UK, this type of contraceptive is used by about one in 20 women who appreciate the convenience of not having to remember to take a daily pill.

Barrier methods

The male and female condom, the diaphragm, cap and spermicides all work by simply stopping the ovum and sperm from meeting. These contraceptives are medically safe, instantly reversible, and therefore appropriate for use during the preconception period. If you are using lubricants with a latex barrier, make sure they are safe as oil-based products damage the rubber very quickly.

Fertility awareness (also called natural family planning: NFP) is another good form of contraception as you prepare for pregnancy because, as well as being free of medical side effects and being instantly reversible, it will help you to determine the days you are most likely to conceive once you are ready (see chapter 3). Remember, however, that it takes between three and six months to learn fertility awareness and identify your own fertility pattern, and you should not rely on this method for contraception until you have learned the method thoroughly. Furthermore, if you have any serious health problems to consider, for instance, dangerous exposure to chemicals at work (see chapter 9: Avoiding Environmental Hazards), a course of strong medication to complete, or you are diabetic and need to get your blood sugar levels under control – you will need a highly effective form of contraception until your doctor has given you the all-clear.

Choosing the right method

The summary chart on pages 76–79 outlines the way each contraceptive works, its efficacy, the time it takes for your fertility to return to normal, and the risks to your baby if you conceive accidentally. This will give you the necessary information to help you make an informed decision about which contraceptive is best for you during your preconception period. If you need further advice, however, don't hesitate to consult your doctor.

By using your body's own fertility signals, you can learn to use fertility awareness to avoid conception while you prepare for pregnancy. This is also called natural family planning (NFP). Some couples choose to avoid intercourse during the woman's fertile time while others prefer to use a barrier method such as a condom. It is worth remembering, however, that using a barrier method at your most fertile time involves a higher risk of accidental conception than it does at other times in your cycle. Abstention from intercourse during your fertile period is the only way to be absolutely safe. Using fertility awareness as a way to avoid pregnancy not only has the benefits of being free from chemical side effects, it will also help you to

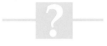

DID YOU KNOW?

Taking the combined oral contraceptive pill may actually help to preserve your fertility – the resulting lack of ovulation helps to protect you from ovarian cysts and endometriosis, the thickening of cervical mucus gives some protection from pelvic inflammatory disease, the hormonal effect on the uterine lining helps to prevent endometrial cancer, and less pregnancies mean less chance of having an ectopic pregnancy!

Contraception the natural way

plan a conception when you and your partner feel the time is right.

Many couples find it daunting having to abstain from sex during the woman's most fertile days. However, learning new ways to give each other pleasure without vaginal intercourse can bring a new dimension to love making. You will appreciate this particularly during pregnancy and the early days after childbirth, when conventional intercourse is not always the most comfortable way to make love. If you feel that it's safest to avoid close sexual contact altogether during your most fertile time, you can

THE PILL AND YOUR FERTILITY

The combined oral contraceptive pill (COC) is a very popular form of contraception, and women thinking of starting a family often wonder when they should stop taking it. Containing oestrogen and a progestagen (synthetic types of progesterone), the pill works by inhibiting ovulation. The "periods" that you get are, in fact, only withdrawal bleeding from the hormones in it. The oestrogen and progestagen maintain the endometrium, and when these hormone levels fall, the endometrium is shed, similar to a natural period, but without ovulation occurring.

Many doctors advise that you stop the pill at least three months before you are ready to conceive. This not only allows your fertility to return to normal (a delay of two to three months is common, although some women ovulate within 10 days), but also allows certain chemicals in your blood to return to normal (the pill alters the blood levels of many vitamins and minerals). On the other hand, some women have a time of increased rebound fertility immediately after stopping the pill, so a long wait may not be advisable.

The delay between stopping the pill and conception rises with age, sometimes up to a year or more for women over 30. If you are in your 30s you may want to consider switching to a more readily reversible form of contraception before you plan to conceive.

After stopping the pill, the fertility awareness techniques described in chapter 3 will help you observe your returning fertility. The first one or two cycles after stopping may not show clear mucus and temperature changes, even if they are in fact fertile. However, as your first ovulation approaches you should begin to notice a change from the dryness or rather sticky mucus caused by the pill to fertile cervical mucus. A sustained temperature rise followed by a period confirms that you are ovulating again. Your natural hormone cycle will allow the build-up of a healthy endometrium and your periods may be heavier. You may also notice Mittelschmerz (abdominal pain) around the time of ovulation.

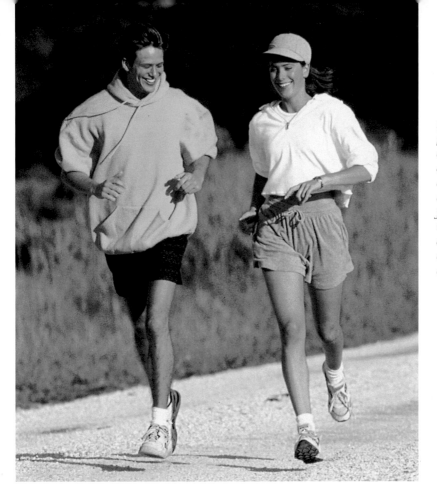

If you and your partner use fertility awareness as a form of contraception and abstain from sex during your most fertile time, take time to enjoy the many other activities you can do together as a couple.

make the most of being able to stay out late and come home too exhausted to make love. These nights will become few and far between when you have small children!

The symptothermal method

If you have learned to chart your periods, cervical mucus, basal body temperature (BBT) and other fertility signs accurately (see chapter 3), you can avoid pregnancy the natural way. Using fertility awareness should be a team effort between both partners, particularly as you may choose to abstain from intercourse at times. Ideally, you should chart at least six cycles to be sure of your own natural variation before you can rely on this method for contraception, although you will begin to see when you are fertile much earlier.

There are two main rules when you use this method to avoid pregnancy. The first is to avoid intercourse as soon as any cervical mucus appears after your period. On the dry days following your period it is usually safe to have intercourse. In practice, it is best to have intercourse on alternate days only so that semen does not mask the appearance of the first cervical mucus, which could nurture sperm for the days leading up to ovulation.

If you have a short cycle, say of 25 days, your cervical mucus may appear straight after your period, so you will have to refrain from intercourse until after you have ovulated. In a long cycle, on the other hand, the cervical mucus may not appear for a week or more. If you have ever had a short menstrual cycle you must assume that your current cycle could be short.

How to calculate the earliest possible fertile day The first possible fertile day is found by subtracting 19 days from your shortest cycle length. This assumes 14 days between ovulation and the next period, and 5 days in which sperm could survive in fertile cervical mucus. For instance, if your shortest menstrual cycle was 25 days, then your first possible fertile day could be day 6 (25 minus 19).

The second rule is to continue avoiding intercourse until after your BBT has been raised for three consecutive days after peak day (the last day of fertile mucus). The post-ovulatory phase of your cycle is infertile, and it starts on the evening of the third recorded raised temperature. Although

A high-flying change

Mary Ann had a busy career as an air hostess and because her work shifts and the changing time zones made taking the pill reliably almost impossible, she had been using injectable hormones as a contraceptive for several years.

"When Jack and I married, I was working on long-haul flights and he was travelling a lot as a company sales rep. After discussing the issue, we agreed it was best to delay starting a family until our lives were a little less hectic and I could find a job on the ground.

About 18 months after our wedding, I started working at the airport in the airline office and Jack and I felt ready to try for a baby. I remember being told by my doctor that my periods would take a while to come back after I stopped having the injections but I was nevertheless very disappointed when I still hadn't had a period six months after my last injection. I talked to my doctor who told me that it could be

another six months or more before I saw regular periods. She reassured me that they would return and suggested that I learn to look out for signs of my returning fertility by learning fertility awareness.

Over the next few months I started noticing patches of mucus on my underwear where I had previously been dry for ages. Then, one day, my temperature went up and two weeks after this I started bleeding. I never thought I'd be so glad to have a period! The next month, Jack returned from a business trip around the 12th day of my cycle and we had intercourse. That month my temperature stayed raised a week after my period was due and a test confirmed that I was pregnant."

the ovum can only survive for 12 to 24 hours, you need to wait three days to be sure that the initial temperature rise is not a "spike" due to illness or a change in routine. Waiting for three consecutive temperature rises also allows for the unlikely event of further ovulation, which could only occur within 24 hours of the first, and allows 24 hours for that ovum to die too.

Your temperature rise should always fit in with your cervical mucus signs. The three raised temperatures should all be after the peak day. If your temperature shift seems to be very early or you are still seeing fertile mucus, wait until the fourth day after the fertile mucus has disappeared before having unprotected intercourse. Remember, if in doubt, wait! You will benefit from an experienced fertility awareness teacher who can lead you through to independence with the method.

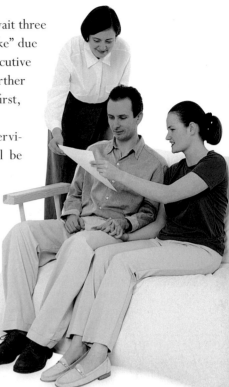

How reliable is this method? No method of contraception is 100 per cent effective and failure rates are made up of two components: method failure (weakness in the method itself) and user failure (where the method isn't used properly). Obviously user failure depends very much on motivation and the accurate use of the method. This is particularly true of natural family planning methods where both partners need to be highly committed to make it work. Indeed, motivation is so important that studies have shown user failure of the symptothermal method as low as one per cent among couples who have completed their family, whereas couples using it merely to space their children are 15 times more likely to conceive accidentally.

Consider spending time with a fertility awareness teacher to learn how to use this method accurately and confidently.

Overall, the theoretical failure rate of this method among well-taught, motivated couples is one to three per cent; in other words, between one and three women out of 100 fall pregnant in a year using this method accurately. This compares well with the condom (two to five per cent) and the progestagen only pill (two per cent). To put it positively, the symptothermal method of contraception is around 97 per cent effective, when used accurately.

Couples who have conceived accidentally using fertility awareness are sometimes concerned about risks to the pregnancy. This stems from the likelihood that conception as a result of intercourse early in a woman's cycle would probably involve an aged sperm, and conception as a result of intercourse after ovulation would probably involve an aged ovum.

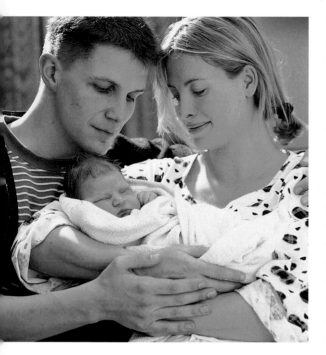

If you conceive accidentally while using fertility awareness as a contraceptive, there is no known health risk to your baby.

However, studies of accidental pregnancies involving fertility awareness have been very reassuring and there is no evidence to suggest health risks to the baby.

The Billings method

This relies on awareness of cervical mucus. Although this method can be used to determine the days you are most likely to be fertile, the Billings method is more often practiced as a way of avoiding pregnancy. To use the Billings method to avoid conception, avoid intercourse from the time your mucus change is first noted after a period, until the fourth day after peak day, which is the last day that fertile mucus is noted. You can have intercourse on alternate dry days after the menstrual period. The restriction to alternate days is because of the possibility of semen masking cervical mucus. Intercourse is unrestricted in the post-ovulatory phase of your cycle.

How reliable is this method? As with the symptothermal method, the Billings method requires careful use. Although failure rates as low as three per cent have been reported, a comparative study of the symptothermal and Billings methods (conducted by M J Wade and published in 1981 in vol 141 of the *American Journal of Obstetrics and Gynecology*) gave a higher failure rate for the Billings method than it did for the symptothermal method. The double check of the basal body temperature to identify the post-ovulatory phase in the symptothermal method gives added safety.

Personal contraceptive system

This computerised system was released in the UK in 1996 and in the US in 1999. It combines information from your previous cycles with urine testing to give a very accurate prediction of your fertile and infertile times. It has been extensively tested in Europe for use as a reliable form of contraception, but it can also be used to help couples predict their fertile time when planning to conceive.

To start programming the device, you will need to log your periods each month and perform a simple dipstick urine test several days each month. The urine test measures a breakdown product of oestrogen to predict that ovulation is approaching and the same urine stick can detect the LH surge. The personal contraceptive displays a red light on fertile days, a green light for infertile days, and an orange light if another urine test is needed. The device is programmed to use the LH surge to determine the end of the fertile time. This is calculated by adding four days, which allows for the expected life of an ovum and the maximum delay of 36 hours from LH surge to ovulation.

How reliable is this method? The personal contraceptive system is 94 per cent effective when used according to its instructions and in conjunction with no other method of contraception, such as a condom or spermicide. Although the device is very easy to use, it is only suitable for women who have regular cycles lasting between 23 and 35 days.

As a contraceptive, the personal contraceptive system is probably less accurate than the symptothermal method in the hands of an experienced user. This is thought to be due to the green light being displayed in the early part of the cycle when, in fact, fertile cervical mucus is beginning to be secreted. As a fertility predictor it is not altogether reliable because relatively infertile days after ovulation would be signalled as "red" or fertile days, when, in fact, you would already notice cervical mucus had dried up, indicating you are not fertile.

TIME TO TALK

Fertility awareness as contraception

If you choose to use fertility awareness as a way to avoid pregnancy, it's very important that you discuss this decision thoroughly with your partner beforehand. You will need to make sure you both understand it well and are fully committed to the restrictions it requires. To help you discuss using fertility awareness as contraception, consider the following questions:

- Will you or your partner feel frustrated and resentful about abstaining from intercourse during the fertile time in your cycle?
- Will your desire for each other increase or decrease during your breaks from lovemaking?
- How will you or your partner feel if your fertile phase falls on a special occasion, such as a birthday or anniversary?
- If you choose to use fertility awareness in conjunction with a barrier method of contraception, will you or your partner find this intrusive? Will either of you be tempted to risk having sex without using it?
- What other activities can you enjoy together as a couple?

CONTRACEPTIVES AND YOUR FERTILITY

The method of contraception you choose while you prepare for pregnancy is very much a matter of personal preference. Understanding how each method works and how it might affect your fertility will help you and your partner to decide which one is best for you during this time. If you need to make a lot of health and lifestyle changes during your preconception period you may want to use a contraceptive that has one of the highest rates of efficacy (that is, the percentage of women who do not conceive during one year of normal use). For example, changes in your eating habits can be made overnight, but if you smoke or are underweight, your body may need a few months to recover from these ill-effects. If you are already in good health you may prefer a contraceptive that has a lower efficacy rate than the others. The efficacy rate of each contraceptive is based on two factors: user failure rate (that is, the method has been used incorrectly) and method failure rate (the contraceptive itself has failed).

HOW IT WORKS	EFFICACY	RETURNING FERTILITY	RISK TO BABY IF CONCEPTION OCCURS
Combined oral contraceptive pill (COC)			
Inhibits ovulation by sending oestrogen and progestagen to the hypothalamus, which then fails to stimulate the pituitary to secrete LH. As a back up, the endometrium does not build up in preparation for conception, and the cervical mucus thickens, which helps prevent sperm from entering the uterus.	99%	Many women ovulate within a few weeks of stopping the pill, some within 10 days. Women over 30 may experience long delays of a year or more and those who have never had a pregnancy seem to experience the longest delays. The fertility of women using the triphasic pills (rather than monophasic pills, which have the same dose throughout each packet) may return more quickly.	Some authorities advise waiting three months after stopping the pill to improve your health, but babies conceived while on or immediately after stopping the pill are not generally affected. Women who conceive accidentally while on the pill and carry on taking it are more likely to have a multiple pregnancy, although twins are less commonly conceived after a woman stops taking the pill.
Progestagen only pills (POP)			
Thickens the cervical mucus to prevent sperm entering the uterus, may inhibit ovulation in some women, interferes with sperm transport in the Fallopian tubes.	98% (probably higher in women over 35)	The contraceptive effect of the POP is very short-lived and fertility may return within 12 hours of a missed dose. There is no evidence to suggest any delay in fertility after using the POP.	Some women on the POP have very infrequent periods, so it's possible to conceive and not realise it. The dose of progestagen in the POP is very low and there is no evidence to suggest that taking the POP by mistake in early pregnancy can damage the baby. However, a higher proportion of POP accidental pregnancies are ectopic. This is probably because the progestagen interferes with the transport of the fertilised ovum in the Fallopian tubes.

HOW IT WORKS	EFFICACY	RETURNING FERTILITY	RISK TO BABY IF CONCEPTION OCCURS

Post-coital contraceptive pills (emergency contraception)

These pills contain a high dose of oestrogen and progestagen and, if taken up to 72 hours after unprotected sexual intercourse, they can disrupt the endometrium and prevent implantation of the fertilised ovum. They can delay the release of an ovum if taken before ovulation.	About 95%	The hormones in these pills usually affect your body only for a few days, so they should have no consequences on your long-term fertility. You could conceive during your next menstrual cycle or even later in the same cycle, although it is advisable to wait for a natural period before attempting to conceive.	A UK national register of pregnancies after failed emergency contraception reported that out of 119 pregnancies, 115 babies were born healthy. Of the few babies with a major abnormality 4 out of the 5 mothers smoked and one was taking a drug known to cause foetal damage. Because this contraception works before any of the baby's organs are formed, the effect is probably "all or nothing," that is, if your pregnancy goes to term, you will most likely have a healthy baby.

Injectable hormones

An intramuscular, slow-release injection of progestagen is given every 2 or 3 months. The amount of progestagen is high enough to inhibit the hypothalamus and pituitary, so very little LH and FSH are released, thus preventing the ovaries from being stimulated. Any cervical mucus produced is infertile.	At least 99%	On average, fertility returns within 6 months of the last dose expiring, but can take up to 18 months, even if you have had only one injection. Not a good method for short-term contraception or for older women wanting to conceive in the near future.	Because it is so effective, very few accidental pregnancies occur and there is very little research on the outcome of these pregnancies. There doesn't seem to be a risk of ectopic pregnancy or miscarriage, although babies may tend to be underweight at birth. This effect is most marked if the baby was exposed to an injection soon after conception.

Subdermal progestagen implants

Six matchstick-sized rods are implanted under the skin of the upper arm and soon a single rod will be available. The rods release progestagen for up to five years, which thickens the cervical mucus and may stop ovulation from occurring in some women.	99.7%	Fertility returns very quickly after removal. About 1 in 5 women ovulate within 4 weeks of its removal, and most by 7 weeks. Although a woman may ovulate again quite quickly, fertility may be delayed as the cervical mucus takes longer to recover. About 80% of women will conceive within a year of stopping.	Because it is so effective, very few accidental pregnancies occur and there is very little research on the outcome of these pregnancies, although the risks should be as low as for the POP.

How it works	Efficacy	Returning fertility	Risk to baby if conception occurs

The intrauterine device (IUD)

Modern devices have a flexible plastic frame wound with copper, which causes a slight inflammatory reaction in the uterus and makes it unreceptive to a fertilised ovum. Sperm motility is also inhibited. A frameless copper intrauterine implant is also available.	Over 99%	Usually immediately. It can cause heavy periods, so blood should be checked for anaemia before trying to conceive. Pelvic infection may be more severe for women using an IUD, so it's preferable not to use an IUD until after you have completed your family.	Accidental pregnancy does not seem to put a baby at risk of developing congenital abnormalities. However, if an IUD is left in place after accidental conception there is more than a 50% risk that the pregnancy will end in miscarriage. If the IUD is removed within the first 3 months of pregnancy, however, there is a high chance of a successful pregnancy.

The intrauterine system (IUS)

This progestagen impregnated IUD combines the effects of the IUD and other progestagen contraceptive methods. Cervical mucus is thickened and impenetrable to sperm so fertilisation is unlikely. If fertilisation occurs, implantation is unlikely. Ovulation may be inhibited and periods usually become light.	99.9%	Fertility should return within weeks after removal. The risk of pelvic infection is reduced due to the progestagenic effect on the cervical mucus, which provides a barrier to any infection.	Because the IUS is so effective there have been very few accidental pregnancies. In the event of an accidental conception, the risk to the baby is likely to be very low. Ectopic pregnancy rates are low and this system is suitable for women who have suffered an ectopic pregnancy before.

Barrier methods (male and female condom, diaphragm, cervical cap) and spermicides

Barrier methods prevent sperm from entering the cervical canal and spermicides kill sperm.	95–8% (in conjunction); 85% (spermicide alone).	Immediately.	Research has shown no increased risk to babies conceived accidentally using barrier methods with spermicides.

Fertility awareness (FA) or natural family planning (NFP)

By learning to recognise the body's fertility signals, you can determine when you ovulate, and avoid intercourse during your fertile times. For further information see chapter 3: Learning Fertility Awareness	97%, if used correctly.	Immediately. May even promote fertility by allowing intercourse to be timed for the fertile days in the menstrual cycle.	Pregnancy may have resulted from aged sperm if conception occurred early in the cycle, or an aged ovum if conception occurred after ovulation. However, recent studies have been very reassuring and there is no evidence to suggest any health risks to a baby conceived accidentally.

HOW IT WORKS	EFFICACY	RETURNING FERTILITY	RISK TO BABY IF CONCEPTION OCCURS

Lactational amenorrhoea method (breast-feeding)

When you breast-feed, the hormone prolactin is released from the pituitary gland. Prolactin inhibits oestrogen production, which means the hypothalamus and pituitary do not send out the surge of LH that stimulates ovulation.	98% if baby is less than 6 months old and is fully breast-fed.	Some women ovulate while breast-feeding, particularly if they are weaning. Others don't ovulate for months after stopping. Half of breast-feeding women ovulate for the first time before the appearance of their first period after the birth.	There is no particular risk to a baby conceived accidentally while you are still breast-feeding except for the disadvantages of close spacing (see page 55). The breast-feeding baby may go off the breast due to a change in the taste of the milk.

Vasectomy (male sterilisation)

The vas deferens is cut in a minor operation (usually under local anaesthetic). The operation takes effect after about 3 months or 30 ejaculations, when all the remaining sperm in the vas deferens have cleared.	99.9 % (In 0.1% of men, that is, 1 in 1,000 men, tubes can rejoin up to several years later.)	Reversal is possible but does not guarantee restored fertility. There is a 90% success rate if reversal is within 2 years and a 50% chance of restored fertility if it's reversed within 10 years. Sperm production may be poor afterwards if the epididymis is damaged from years of obstruction and distension. About 60% of men develop antibodies to their own sperm afterward and this can prevent fertilisation.	Accidental conception after vasectomy would either be due to failure or natural reversal. It is not known whether there is a risk to such pregnancies, but in theory they should be healthy.

Tubal ligation (female sterilisation)

The Fallopian tubes are cut or clipped in a short operation, usually under general anaesthetic. This means that ovum and sperm can never meet. A tubal ligation is effective immediately.	Over 99% (Failure rates of 1 in 200–300 have recently been reported in the US.)	Tubes can be reunited using microsurgery. Success depends on the skill of the surgeon and the original operation technique used. Reversal is twice as likely to be successful if a woman is under 35. One in 300 women becomes fertile again without a reversal, even many years later, because the tubes can regrow and attach to each other again.	The chances of having an ectopic pregnancy are increased after a sterilisation reversal because the tubes may remain distorted or damaged, but there is no risk to the baby if the pregnancy is normal.

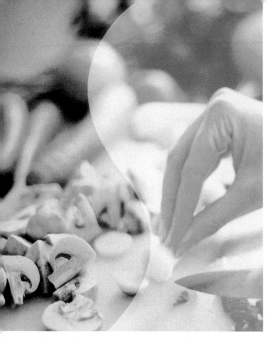

Food For Fertility

Every day we are bombarded by messages about the food we eat and, as so many of them seem to be conflicting, it's easy to feel confused. Yet eating healthily doesn't have to be complicated. Establishing a proper diet now will improve your fertility and lay the foundation for good nutrition during pregnancy, as well as at the family dinner table in the years to come. What's more, a healthy diet will help both you and your partner to improve your physical fitness in preparation for the demanding role of parenthood.

Why diet matters

If you are reading this book you are almost certainly among the world's fortunate who have easy access to a choice of supermarkets filled with a wide variety of fresh and attractive foods. You are also most likely to have a refrigerator and freezer at home for the safe storage of this food. Yet with so many quick and cheap convenience foods at our disposal, the quality of the modern-day diet is often well below par. Numerous consumer surveys demonstrate that, regardless of income, many men and women do not eat any fresh fruits or vegetables each day. Because many vitamins and minerals are lost when fresh food is refined, heated and stored, it's very important that you fill your diet with a wide variety of food types – particularly fresh vegetables and fruits – so that you provide your body with the vitamins, minerals and other ingredients essential for its healthy function. In fact, vitamins are so named because they are vital to life.

The earlier the better

Perhaps you have promised yourself that once you are pregnant you will improve your diet, but it is just as important to improve your diet before you conceive. This is because the cells in a baby's body are most vulnerable to the effects of poor nutrition when they are dividing and most of this cell division takes place during the early weeks of pregnancy, sometimes before a woman even knows she is pregnant. The much-publicised research on the vitamin known as folic acid (see page 89) indicates that taking extra folic acid before you conceive and during early pregnancy will help with the development of your baby's nervous system and reduce the risk of spina bifida. Starting to take it once you know you are pregnant may be too late.

The importance of a good preconception diet was well illustrated by the research undertaken on children born during annual food shortages in The Gambia. Climatic conditions in this sub-Saharan African country meant that crops could only be harvested once a year, and this led to a long, "hungry" season when food was in short supply. In 1950, Professor Sir Ian McGregor (then a young scientist) initiated a painstaking study which revealed that women who were pregnant during the hungry season suffered considerable malnutrition and weight loss. This, in turn, caused their babies' development in utero to be significantly retarded. Furthermore, these babies had a poor life expectancy in adulthood compared to babies born after the harvest, suggesting that lifelong resistance to infection is programmed at birth.

IN UTERO AND FOREVER AFTER

The relationship between diet and a healthy pregnancy has been well documented, but recent research in the UK's Southampton University by Professor David Barker has revealed that the nourishment a baby receives in the uterus not only affects his health at the time of birth, but also his health as an adult. If a woman has not been well nourished during her pregnancy, the chances of her baby developing high blood pressure, ischaemic heart disease and diabetes all increase. Female fertility also can be affected at this early stage, and baby girls who are poorly nourished in utero may themselves go on to give birth to low birth-weight babies. This means that being careful with your diet before you conceive and during early pregnancy may even help to safeguard the health of your future grandchildren!

Dad's diet

Maternal diet is not the only contributing factor to your baby's healthy development. Animal breeders are fully aware of the importance of the male diet for good fertility, yet very little attention is paid to the human male diet when thinking about fertility and successful conception. Deficiencies in many vitamins and minerals have been shown to affect fertility in animals and this applies to humans too: it is now well known that vitamins A, B complex and the minerals magnesium, zinc and selenium are all-important in the processes of male fertility. But before you or your partner rush out to buy supplements, remember that a well-balanced diet is usually the safest way for men and women to improve their vitamin and mineral intake (unless specific deficiencies are being corrected), as high doses of many minerals and vitamins are known to be toxic (see page 96).

Even a temporary lapse in diet, for instance, during a one- or two-week bout of flu can affect semen quality. So, after a period of poor diet, men should allow at least three to four months – the time needed for the formation and ejaculation of new, healthy sperm – before they attempt to conceive.

The essentials for a healthy diet

A healthy diet provides you with all the energy and building materials that your body needs each day. To ensure that you are in optimum health for fertility, conception and pregnancy, you need to eat a variety of foods from each of the main food groups each day. These groups consist of carbohydrates or starchy foods; fruits and vegetables; protein-rich foods such as nuts, meat, eggs and dairy products; and fats or oils (needed only in small amounts). Both quantity and quality is important, and the following pages will help you to eat well for fertility. If you are unsure whether your current diet is adequate, why not keep a record of the foods you eat for a couple of weeks, which will help you keep track of your nutrient intake.

Carbohydrates

Starchy foods such as bread, potatoes, rice, cereals and pasta are energy-rich and should form the foundation of a healthy diet. They are also major sources of vital nutrients. For example, wholemeal bread, wholegrain cereals and brown rice all provide iron and vitamin B complex. However, it's important that you eat these foods in their most natural form. Many refined or "white" versions have lost much of their natural vitamins and minerals, although some refined flours are fortified to add back some of the lost nutrients.

As you start to improve your diet and adopt a healthier lifestyle in preparation for conception and pregnancy, try to cut down on processed, sugary snacks and choose foods like bananas, corn on the cob, or brown rice cakes when you need an energy boost. These starchy energy sources are naturally low in fat, yet high in vitamins and fibre, which helps to release their energy slowly, as you need it. Snacks that are made from more refined carbohydrates, such as boiled sweets or white bread, will not

Starting the day right

In today's busy world, it's easy to skip having a proper breakfast. But even though it may be the smallest meal of your day, it should be no less important than any of the other meals you have. An energy-rich breakfast, including wholegrain cereal or wholemeal toast, is a great way to boost your nutrient intake and improve your health for conception and beyond.

A survey into the eating habits of a group of pregnant women in London (Wendy Doyle, 1982) showed that those who gave birth to large, healthy babies ate twice as much breakfast cereal, wholemeal bread and eggs than those who delivered underweight babies.

have as many nutrients and will not satisfy your appetite for as long.

Fibre

Also known as roughage, fibre is not digested but instead remains in the bowel where it helps the intestines to propel waste products effortlessly along. This ensures that energy is steadily absorbed, fat absorption is controlled, and our bodies are protected from the effects of toxins. Low-fibre diets tend to cause constipation, haemorrhoids, an increased risk of colon cancer and raised cholesterol levels (which are associated with heart disease). Making sure you have enough fibre in your diet is therefore particularly important while you are pregnant, when slower bowel muscle activity may leave you prone to constipation or haemorrhoids.

All fruits and vegetables are valuable sources of fibre, as are wheat, rice, wholemeal cereals and nuts. However, it is much better to get your fibre from fresh sources rather than from refined ones (bran, for example) as eating refined fibre may actually prevent you from absorbing some minerals.

Fruits and vegetables

Modern cultivation, transport and refrigeration methods now mean that there is a wide variety of fruits and vegetables all year round, yet it is easy to end up eating the same few varieties week after week. Although all fruits and vegetables are sources of energy and fibre, the vitamin and mineral contents vary widely and this is why you should try to include a good variety in your diet. Citrus fruits, for instance, are good sources of vitamin C but are not particularly rich in folic acid. Red and orange vegetables including tomatoes, carrots and peppers are good sources of vitamin A, but carrots contain very little vitamin C. The chart on pages 92–95 will help you choose which vegetables and fruits to eat to boost your intake of specific vitamins and minerals.

Keeping the goodness in You can increase your vitamin and mineral intake just by the way you prepare your food. Many of the nutrients found in vegetables are destroyed by heat and storage, so it's best to eat many of them raw and as fresh as possible.

HEALTHY SPERM AND OVA

Some foods have being shown to contain powerful protective substances called antimutagens (the vitamins A, C, and E are known antimutagens). These help to protect us from developing cancer and are also likely to help prevent genetic defects in rapidly dividing sperm cells and ova. In 1978, scientists from the Japanese Institute of Genetics tested 59 fruits and vegetables and almost all were found to counteract poisons which damage dividing cells (mutagens). Among the best were mint leaves, parsley, ginger, garlic, shallots, broccoli, green peppers, cabbage, cauliflower and pineapple.

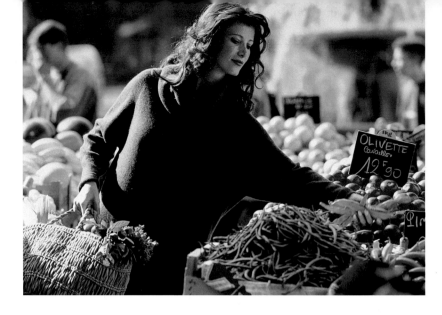

Fruits and vegetables come in an almost infinite variety of colours, shapes and forms, so be adventurous and try to purchase different types each week.

When you cook vegetables, light steaming or quick stir-frying (rather than boiling) helps to preserve nutrients – and never presoak vegetables. Avoid reheating food, which will destroy vitamins even further. If you boil vegetables, many of the nutrients (such as vitamins B6 and C) will leach out into the water, so use any liquid from cooking for sauces, stocks and soups. Don't add bicarbonate of soda to keep the colour of green vegetables as this destroys vitamins B1, B2 and B5.

Most fruits and vegetables start to lose their vitamins the minute they are picked – for example, a third of a product's vitamin C may be lost in a day – which makes homegrown or freshly harvested vegetables the best choice. Surprisingly, frozen vegetables are often better for you than fresh vegetables that are stored for days in a shop, because many are processed and frozen within hours of harvesting. When you need to store vegetables, refrigerate them as soon as you bring them home and don't wash them until necessary. Keep cutting and chopping to a minimum or do this just before serving because enzymes released at the cut surface will start to break down vitamins. Because many vitamins lie just under the skin of fruit and vegetables, you should only peel where absolutely necessary. Peeling is sometimes advised if foods have been treated with pesticides because the pollutants then lie in the skin. Home or organically grown fruits and vegetables can be eaten unpeeled.

Products that contain vitamin A (such as carrots, spring greens and tomatoes) and vitamin C (apples and potatoes) also will need to be stored in dark places because their nutrients are destroyed by light.

Proteins

Meat, fish, eggs, dairy products, pulses and nuts are all major sources of protein, a nutrient that is important for the growth and repair of the human body, and therefore vital for the growth of a developing baby. Beans and pulses are also good sources of energy and are high in fibre too. Wholegrain cereals also contain valuable protein, as well as starch. Nuts are particularly good snacks because they are rich in a variety of vitamins and minerals, such a vitamin E and magnesium. They do have a higher fat content than pulses, however, so should be eaten in moderation. Dried beans and pulses require soaking and long cooking times, but many are available precooked in cans. If you are going to rely heavily on them for your protein, bear in mind that they often contain added salt and sugar. Canned baked beans are a prime example.

Because different protein sources vary in the amount of other nutrients they contain, it's important that you eat a wide variety. Foods rich in vegetable protein, such as beans, pulses and grains, usually contain plenty of fibre, energy and vitamins, but may be low in iron and lack vitamin B12. Moreover, although red meat and eggs are high in protein and iron, they also can contain high levels of saturated fat (see page 86).

For vegetarians and vegans If you choose to exclude animal products from your diet, take care to include a wide variety of foods, especially protein sources. If you are the only vegetarian in your household make sure you substitute meat with pulses, beans, wholegrain cereals and dairy products instead of just leaving the meat part out of each meal. If you are on a vegan diet and don't eat any foods derived from animals (including milk and eggs) you also may be lacking in vitamin B12 as this vitamin is almost exclusively found in animal products. The exceptions are fortified cereals, certain seaweeds and yeast extract, so make sure your diet includes some of these foods. Some fortified foods use B12 from animal foods, but synthetic supplements acceptable for a vegan diet do exist.

Dairy products

These foods are all derived from milk and form an important part of the Western diet, especially as a source of calcium (see page 90), magnesium (see page 95) and riboflavin (see page 92). Milk-derived products, such as cheese and yoghurt, can also be an important source of protein for vegetarians.

Although many of us rely on milk products for our calcium intake, there are other non-dairy sources, such as sardines, spinach and wholegrain flours. Full-fat milk products, butter and hard cheeses are high in cholesterol and other saturated fats (which you may need to cut down on), so choose low-fat milk, yoghurts and cheeses which contain the same amount of calcium but are lower in fat and cholesterol. Completely

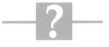

DID YOU KNOW?

It's been known for centuries that some substances in foods prevent diseases. Nicknamed Limeys, British sailors in the late 18th century took fresh limes on sea voyages to prevent scurvy, a disease caused by vitamin C deficiency. However, it wasn't until 1912 that the first vitamin was chemically isolated and named "vitamin A" (short for vital amine). As each new vitamin was identified it was assigned a new letter of the alphabet. Vitamin B, the second to be discovered, was subsequently found to be a whole group of substances, hence the numbers B1, B2 and so on.

Try visualising a healthy, balanced diet as a pyramid of food. This will help you decide the proportion of different foods to eat in your diet.

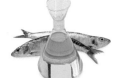

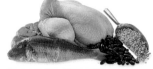

Oils and fats: Eat oily fish 1–2 times a week and use vegetable oils.

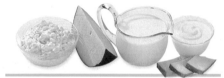

Proteins: 2 portions a day is ample. A portion = 3 oz meat, 4 oz fish, or 5 oz cooked lentils or beans.

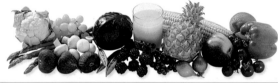

Dairy products: If this is your main source of calcium eat 3 portions of low fat varieties a day. A portion = ⅓ pint of milk, 5 oz yoghurt, 40 g cheese.

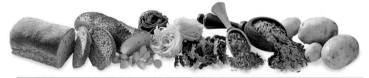

Fruits and vegetables: Aim for 5 portions a day. If you eat enough, fibre should take care of itself. A portion = glass of orange juice, 1 large piece of fruit, 3 tablespoons of cooked vegetables.

Carbohydrates: These should form the largest component of your diet. Eat 4 to 6 portions a day, depending on appetite and exercise levels. A portion = 2 slices of bread, 5 oz potatoes, 4 tablespoons cooked rice, 6 tablespoons cooked pasta.

skimmed milk is also available, but it is important to note that the fat soluble vitamins A and D are lost in skimmed milk (although some manufacturers add them back). Certain nutrients in milk, such as vitamins B2, B3 and B12, are also destroyed by light so make sure you don't leave milk out of the refrigerator for too long.

Oils and fats

Butter, margarine and cooking oil are all obvious sources of fat in our diet, but other foods such as dairy products, meat, fish, nuts and even wholegrains contain fats as well. Our bodies can use fat for energy but if we eat too much of it, we store it in the all too familiar places because it cannot be excreted as waste. If your calorie intake matches up to the amount you burn every day, you may not put on weight, but watch out: if too many calories come from fat, you will be short of the vitamins and fibre that you would get if your calories came mostly from starchy foods and vegetables. You should aim to get no more than a third of your calories from fat and as few as possible from saturated fats.

There are three kinds of fat in our diet: saturated, monounsaturated and polyunsaturated, but only the polyunsaturates are essential. These are vital for the production of sex hormones such as testosterone, oestrogen, and progesterone. Saturated fats are found in meat, lard, butter and margarine (and therefore in pies, cakes and biscuits) and tend to be hard fats that are thought to be partly responsible for the high incidence of heart disease in Western countries. Monounsaturated fats, found in plant oils such as olive oil, peanut oil, sun-

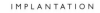

flower oil and avocados, are a safer option, even possibly helping to prevent heart disease.

The essential polyunsaturated fats are linoleic and linolenic acids. Linoleic acid is found in sunflower, corn, soya, evening primrose, starflower and blackcurrant oils, and linolenic acid is found in oily fish such as herring, salmon and mackerel. The oils in these foods are often good sources of the fat-soluble vitamins (A, D, E and K).

Salt

In small amounts, salt is essential as it helps to maintain fluid balance and many other aspects of body function. However, the average Western diet contains three or four times more salt than necessary, which puts a strain on the kidneys. The jury is still out on the precise effects of salt on blood pressure and heart disease, but as high salt intake does seem to be a cause of high blood pressure, it is important to reduce your salt intake to healthy levels before pregnancy, when high blood pressure becomes very danger-ous. If you tend to sprinkle salt liberally over everything you eat, bear in mind that as a general rule, a varied diet will naturally contain enough salt without the need to add any. And watch out for hidden sources of excess salt in processed foods, cured meats, cheeses and some bread.

Vitamins are essential chemicals that we need for vital processes through-out our bodies but which we cannot manufacture ourselves. Minerals are also necessary in every cell of our bodies for chemical reactions, bone structure and fluid balance. Our bodies contain most of the minerals found on the planet and many are essential to life. Some minerals are found so widely in food that we are unlikely to become deficient. Others, such as the metals cadmium and lead, are toxic and don't appear naturally in food-stuffs except as a result of pollution. We need only very small amounts (by weight) of vitamins and minerals, and sometimes too much is just as harmful as too little.

We are mostly dependent on food sources for our intake of the numerous vitamins and minerals, which is why diet is so important for good health. The chart on pages 92–95 indicates the functions of each vitamin or mineral, and how to boost your dietary intake without resorting to supplements. As mentioned earlier, many vitamins and minerals are quite fragile, and are easily destroyed by heat, storage, and sometimes light (especially the B vitamins). Consequently, nutrient-rich fruits and vegeta-bles are usually best eaten raw and as fresh as possible.

DID YOU KNOW?

Most margarines that are made from liquid vegetable oils are often advertised as being healthy because the origi-nal oil contains polyunsat-urated fat. However, when liquid vegetable oil is processed and becomes more solid, some of the fats in the oil are changed into substances called trans-fatty acids. These may be as harmful as saturated fats and have been linked to heart disease. Therefore, where possible, always try to use naturally liquid oils, such as olive oil and other vegetable oils.

Vitamins and minerals

Boosting your intake before and during pregnancy

If you are already eating a broad range of foods and consuming the recommended daily allowance (RDI) of all the nutrients necessary for a healthy adult diet, then you probably won't need to change your eating habits very much during your preconception period (for more information see Looking Ahead on page 100). However, there are some vitamins and minerals that are particularly important at this time and you may need to boost your intake of these if you are trying for a baby or are already pregnant.

Folic acid Until recently, folic acid was just another B complex vitamin, but now conclusive research has shown its vital role in the prevention of spina bifida. It has been known for many years that women who have already had a baby with a neural tube defect, such as spina bifida or anencephaly, are more likely than other women to face this tragedy again. In the 1960s and 1970s, scientists began to show that multivitamins and an improved diet rich in vegetables seemed to reduce the risk in most mothers. As a result, a detailed research project on over 1,800 pregnancies in the UK and other European countries known to be at high risk of spina bifida was commissioned by the Medical Research Council to confirm which vitamin was protective. The results, published in 1991, showed that of the women who took a folic acid supplement before conception and in early pregnancy, over 70 per cent of expected neural tube defects (i.e., defects affecting a baby's spinal cord and brain) were prevented.

Instead of taking a supplement, it's possible for women planning a pregnancy to get the recommended daily intake of folic acid (600 mcg) through a diet of folate-rich foods.

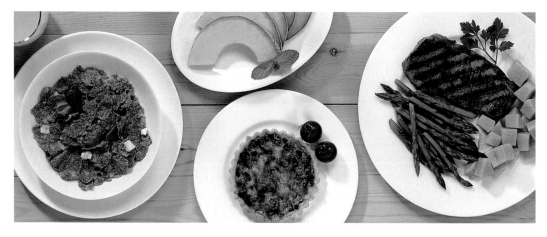

A bowl of fortified cereal and a glass of orange juice at breakfast provide approximately 150 mcg of folic acid.

A spinach and cheese quiche and a large segment of cantaloupe for lunch provide approximately 300 mcg of folic acid.

Sirloin steak with pumpkin and asparagus for dinner provide approximately 200 mcg of folic acid.

Preventing spina bifida

Jackie and Brian experienced the heart-breaking discovery that their unborn baby was affected by spina bifida; he was later stillborn. After a few months, they decided to seek the advice of their doctor before they tried for another baby.

"When we were expecting our first baby, a routine scan at 18 weeks indicated that he had a poorly developed brain and spina bifida. Not only were we completely shocked, we also had to face the agonising decision of whether to proceed with the pregnancy or not. In the end nature took care of the situation and our baby was stillborn shortly afterwards.

Because the whole experience had been so traumatic, I couldn't bear to think about having another baby for a long while. However, time is a great healer and after a few months I felt able to contemplate getting pregnant again. I went to see my doctor, who explained that the risk of having a baby with neural tube defects, such as spina bifida, can be greatly reduced by taking folic acid. She advised us to improve our diets, eating more green, leafy vegetables, and told me I should start taking a folic acid supplement.

Four months after following this advice, Brian and I decided to take the plunge. It took a few months before I finally conceived and our reaction to this pregnancy was much more guarded than last time.

The results of all the blood tests and early scans seemed to indicate that the baby would be fine, but even so, you can imagine how relieved we were when Lucy was finally born and we could actually hold her and see how healthy she was."

In other research centres around the world, such as in Australia and the US, studies were also indicating that low-risk mothers could also reduce their risk of having a baby affected by spina bifida if they increased their folic acid intake not only in early pregnancy, but also from before the moment of conception. (As a result, both the US and the UK governments have now issued guidelines recommending increased folic acid intake for all women planning a pregnancy.)

The average folic acid intake for Western women is around 240 micrograms (mcg) a day, but varies from 80 to 1,000 mcg depending on the kinds of foods that are included in their diet. This is adequate for most adults, but women planning a pregnancy are now advised to increase their intake to around 600 mcg a day either through eating folate-rich foods (see meal plan on page 88) or by taking a 400 mcg supplement. Folic acid supplements are now widely and cheaply available. It's important to remember that you need to increase your folic acid from before the time you conceive and continue until at least the 12th week of your pregnancy. By this time, your baby's nervous system will be well developed.

If you have already had a baby affected by a neural tube defect, or if you or a close relative has been affected, you will need to take a larger sup-

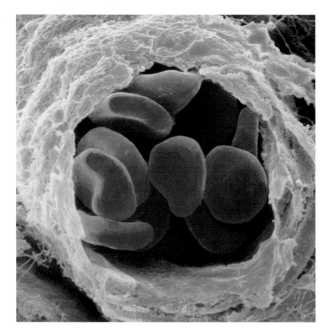

Red blood cells (seen below) contain haemoglobin, a vital substance that carries oxygen around the body. Haemoglobin requires iron for its formation.

plement of 5,000 mcg a day. This can be provided by your doctor or family planning clinic on prescription.

Iron Many women of childbearing age suffer a shortage of this mineral because of heavy blood loss during menstruation, as well as poor diet. The RDI for iron is around 15 mg for all women, and although you and your baby will need a bit more iron during pregnancy, the RDI doesn't rise because absorption of iron improves during pregnancy and there is no loss from menstruation. Your body can store iron, so take a good look at your iron intake before you conceive and boost your iron stores.

It's always better to get your iron from food rather than a supplement, as these can result in unpleasant heartburn and constipation (which are common enough problems in pregnancy without this additional cause). Remember, however, to eat iron with foods rich in vitamin C, as this aids the body's absorption of iron (add tomatoes to a meat casserole, for example). For good sources of iron refer to the chart on pages 92–95.

Calcium Sufficient calcium intake is particularly important throughout pregnancy when your growing baby is developing his or her skeleton. If you do not have enough calcium in your diet during pregnancy, your baby poaches calcium from your own bones, which could leave your bones thinner and your teeth at risk of decay. An adequate supply of calcium during pregnancy may also help to reduce the risk of pre-eclampsia (see page 159).

In pregnancy, boost your calcium intake by eating an extra portion a day, for example, ⅓ pint of milk, a slice of cheese or a helping of yoghurt. You can also make your own "supersource" by boiling up bones into a stock, including a teaspoon of vinegar to leach out the calcium and adding herbs to taste.

Selenium This is used to form selenoproteins, antioxidants that protect the body from the harmful effects of free radicals that damage cell membranes and the delicate processes of cell division. Although we need only very small amounts of it (the RDI is about 75 mcg), selenium is essential for the production of healthy sperm with strong tails. Low levels in men are often associated with low sperm counts and immotile sperm. In women, selenium deficiency has been linked with miscarriage, but the cause is not fully understood.

We rely entirely on food for our intake of selenium but the amount of selenium in foods depends on where it is grown. Over the last 20 years, selenium intakes have been falling in Europe and this is thought to be due to the switch from eating foods made from selenium-rich North American flour to foods made from relatively deficient European flour. Acid rain and other environmental factors have caused soils to become selenium deficient. Finland is one country that has overcome this problem by adding selenium-rich fertiliser to the soil.

Zinc Although our bodies contain only small amounts of zinc, it is lost in sweat and urine so a daily supply is necessary. Zinc is required for growth and tissue repair and is vital in the development of unborn babies. Women who are zinc-deficient during pregnancy tend to have underweight babies who may struggle to thrive in the early weeks after birth. Zinc requirements do rise in pregnancy but if you are already getting enough, your body will adapt by increasing its absorption. Zinc is also important for male reproductive function. It is an antioxidant that protects sperm and is also an important component of semen as it may help the enzymes in the acrosome tip (the head of the sperm) penetrate the ovum at the right time for fertilisation. This may be why oysters, an excellent source of zinc, have long been associated with romance.

Most professionals agree that we should aim to get the vitamins and minerals we need from a healthy diet before reaching for a supplement. But if your diet is poor, perhaps because you have a food allergy or illness or you are experiencing nausea in early pregnancy, you could consider taking a balanced multivitamin and mineral preparation which has been passed as safe for pregnancy. A balanced preparation should only contain each vitamin and mineral at the recommended daily allowance. Folic acid is an exception and all women considering a pregnancy are recommended to take a supplement of 400 mcg before conception and during the first three months of pregnancy, as the average woman would find it difficult to increase her intake sufficiently. However, it is possible to obtain adequate quantities from your diet (see also page 88).

Supplements: who needs them?

ESSENTIAL VITAMINS AND MINERALS

The recommended daily allowance (RDI) is usually the minimum required to prevent deficiency diseases. More is some-times advisable before and during pregnancy, but be careful not to overdose with supplements. The RDI is measured by weight – 1 milligram (mg) = 1,000 micrograms (mcg). The "superfoods" are particularly rich in each nutrient and can be eaten safely without risk of overdose. The percentage of RDI in a portion of superfood is indicated in the chart.

FUNCTION	SOURCES AND SUPERFOODS	COOKING AND STORAGE	DANGERS FROM EXCESS
Vitamin A (also called retinol) RDA = 600 mcg; 700 mcg in pregnancy			
For growth, healthy skin, resistance to infection and night vision. Also made by the body using betac-arotene from plant sources.	Retinol: egg yolk, butter, milk and oily fish. Betacarotene: red, orange and green vegetables, e.g. carrots. 1 sweet potato: 150 g = 150%	Can be destroyed by high temperatures and light so avoid frying and store in the dark. Is also fat soluble and is lost when milk is skimmed.	More than 4 times the RDI of retinol from animal products (liver and kidneys) may cause birth defects so avoid during pregnancy. Betacarotene is safe so you can't overdose.
Vitamin B1 (also called thiamine) RDA = 0.4 mg per 1,000 calories of food			
To convert starchy foods into energy. This is why the RDI is in proportion to carbohydrate intake.	Wholegrain cereals (major energy sources), meat, yeast extract, dairy pro-duce, eggs, and many veg-etables. Peas: 75 g = c.20% (for 2,500 cals) Jacket potato: 1 = c.300%	Lost when grains are milled (ie in bread, refined sugar and white rice). Leaches into cooking water so use this for sauces, soups and stocks. Destroyed by bicar-bonate or baking soda.	Unlikely, because the more starch you eat the more you need.
Vitamin B2 (also called riboflavin) RDA = 1.1 mg; 1.4 mg in pregnancy			
To use energy and keep skin and eyes healthy.	Meat, dairy produce, cere-als, some fruits and vegeta-bles. Kidneys (50 g = 100%) Milk (1/2 pint = 50%)	Lost when grains are milled. Although it leaches out into cooking water it is not destroyed, so use all vegetable water for sauces, stocks and soups.	Unlikely, because the more energy you use, the more vitamin B2 you need.
Vitamin B3 (also called niacin) RDA = 6.6 mg per 1,000 calories, or approximately 15 mg per day			
For energy production.	Fish, meat, nuts, whole-grains. Tuna (90 g = 100%)	Lost when grains are milled. Use vegetable water for stock.	Deficiency is more likely as vitamin B3 is easily lost in cooking liquids.

FUNCTION	SOURCES AND SUPERFOODS	COOKING AND STORAGE	DANGERS FROM EXCESS
Vitamin B6 (also called pyridoxine) RDA = 15 mcg per gram of protein			
To help build new tissues and produce healthy red blood cells. Deficiency can cause anaemia.	Our intestinal bacteria provide some and the rest comes from fruit, vegetables, meat and fish. Cooked lentils: 1 cup = 50% Watermelon: 1 large slice = 50% Avocado: 1 = 100%	Although it leaches out into cooking water it is not destroyed, so use all vegetable water for sauces, stocks and soups.	B6 has become popular for its possible relief of PMS, but can be dangerous in excess. Over 2,000 mcg a day can cause nerve damage but overdose is impossible from dietary sources alone.
Vitamin B12 (also called cobalamin) RDA = 1.5 mcg			
Needed by all fast-dividing cells, so especially important during early pregnancy. Deficiency leads to anaemia and damage to nervous system. It may also contribute to some birth defects.	Usually found only in animal products, e.g. meat, fish, eggs and dairy produce. The only plant foods known to contain B12 are some seaweeds. Spirula seaweed 15 g = 100% Sardines: 10 g = 100% Eggs: 1 = 50%	Although it leaches out into cooking water it is not destroyed, so use all vegetable water for sauces, stocks and soups. Destroyed by bicarbonate or baking soda.	Excess from food not likely.
Vitamin C (also called ascorbic acid) RDA = 40 mg; 50 mg in pregnancy			
For healthy gums, teeth, bones and skin, and to resist infection. Aids iron absorption. Helps body overcome toxins. Used in hormone production.	Most fruit and vegetables. Citrus fruits, potatoes and green vegetables are particularly good sources. Tinned guava: 1 = 200% Orange: 1 = 200% Green pepper: 1/4 = 100%	Up to 100% can be destroyed in cooking, especially if you boil or presoak vegetables. It is also lost through storing, especially in warmth and light.	Large doses may increase absorption of oestrogens from the pill, so if you suddenly stop taking supplements you may get withdrawal bleeds. No danger of excess from food sources.
Vitamin D (also called calciferol) RDA = 10 mcg			
Used by the body to absorb and metabolise calcium.	Fortified margarine, eggs, oily fish. Can be produced in the skin if it's exposed to sunlight. Grilled herring 1 = 100%	Fat soluble so is lost in fully skimmed milk products. Choose vitamin-enriched foods where the vitamin is added back in.	High levels cause thirst and loss of appetite. Avoid very high doses of fish oils as these may also contain high levels of vitamin A.

FUNCTION	SOURCES AND SUPERFOODS	COOKING AND STORAGE	DANGERS FROM EXCESS
Vitamin E (also known as tocopherol) Needed in proportion to the polyunsaturated (vegetable) fat in diet			
Important antioxidant that helps tissues in the body protect themselves from damage.	Plant oils including sunflower and corn, unrefined wholegrain cereals. Wheatgerm.	Levels drop after three months of freezing. Is also destroyed at frying temperatures.	Overdose impossible from ordinary foods, but high-dose supplements should be avoided in pregnancy.
Folic acid (also called folate) RDA = 200 mcg; 600 mcg during preconception period and pregnancy			
For protein synthesis, formation of red blood cells and cell division. Deficiency can cause neural tube defects.	Leafy green vegetables, wholegrain cereals, yeast extract Black-eye beans: 4 tbs = 220 mcg Orange: 1 = 50 mcg Fortified cereal: 1 bowl = 100 mcg	Although it leaches out into cooking water it is not destroyed, so use all vegetable water for sauces, stocks and soups.	Excess from diet impossible. Best to take supplements in the recommended dose. The higher doses given to high-risk mothers are known to be safe.
Vitamin K RDA = approximately 1 mcg per kg of body weight			
Essential for the healthy clotting of blood.	Leafy green vegetables. Some vitamin K is also made in the intestine by bacteria. Broccoli.	Fat soluble, so unlikely to be lost in cooking water.	Impossible from diet. Some-times supplements are given to newborn babies to prevent bleeding early on.
Calcium RDA = 1,000 mg; 1,200 mg in pregnancy			
For growth and daily maintenance of bones and teeth. Vital for blood clotting, and nerve and cell function.	Dairy products, soy milk, sardines, wholegrain cereals, bread. Milk: 1/3 pint = 25% Yoghurt: 5 oz carton = 25% Whitebait: 2 oz = 50%	Skimmed milk products are as rich in calcium as whole milk products. Cooking does not affect calcium content.	Excess from supplements possible in high doses and can contribute to kidney and gall stones.
Iodine RDA = 140 mcg			
Maintains normal thyroid function, which regulates metabolism. Poor thyroid function can depress ovulation. Vital for developing foetal nervous system.	Seafood, iodized salt, dairy products, eggs. Grilled cod: 4 oz = 100% Iodized salt: 1 pinch = 100% Yoghurt: 1 carton = 50%	Not lost in cooking. It is better, however, to derive your iodine from seaweed and seafoods than to add too much salt to your cooking.	Excess from food not possible.

Function	Sources and superfoods	Cooking and storage	Dangers from excess
Iron RDA = 15 mg			
Vital for production of haemoglobin. Deficiency leads to anaemia.	Red meat, liver, eggs, spinach, pulses. Dried figs: 8 = 30% Beef: 4 oz = 30%	Tannin in tea and coffee binds with iron, preventing its absorption, so avoid drinking these with foods containing iron. Bran has the same effect.	Supplements can cause heartburn and constipation. Food sources (especially animal sources) are better absorbed.
Magnesium RDA = 270 mg; 300 mg for young women under 20 during pregnancy			
Needed to build skeleton and for energy production throughout the body.	Most foods, including dairy products, nuts, vegetables and meat. Cooked brown rice: 4 tbs = 25% Sunflower seeds: 1 oz = 30%	Up to 15% is obtained in tap water, especially in hard-water areas. Content in mineral water varies.	Although high-dose supplements are used to treat PMS, avoid these when trying to conceive and get magnesium from food sources instead.
Potassium RDA = 3,500 mg			
Vital for healthy fluid balance in the body.	All fruit, vegetables, meat, pulses and wholegrains. Avocado: 1 = 30% Banana: 1 = 10%	Potassium salt is a safer, healthier alternative to ordinary cooking salt, which may raise blood pressure.	Not possible from food sources.
Selenium RDA = 60–75 mcg			
Protects body from damage to cell membranes and during cell division. Lack of selenium can lead to infertility in men, and possibly miscarriage in women.	Meat, fish (especially mackerel, kippers and herring), and wholemeal flour. Brazil nuts: 2 = 100% Canned tuna: 4 oz = 100% Foods that are made from	flours originating in North America have higher amounts of selenium than those originating in Europe.	No danger from food sources. High dose supplements can be toxic so increase your intake safely through your diet instead.
Zinc RDA = 7–15 mg			
Needed for growth and tissue repair and is vital in the healthy development of unborn babies.	Meat, seafood, wholegrains and dairy products. Beef: 4–8 oz = 100%	Can be lost after repeated cooking and processing so eat fresh, unprocessed foods.	None.

It has become fashionable to take megadoses (several times the RDI) of single vitamins. For instance, many people take megadoses of vitamin C to keep infections at bay, and some women take vitamin B6 to help relieve the symptoms of PMS. But certain nutrients can be positively dangerous if the RDI is exceeded. Taking a supplement of more than 2,000 mcg of vitamin B6, for example, can cause nerve damage, whereas overdosing on this vitamin via a food source would be impossible.

You should avoid all megadoses of vitamins and minerals when you plan to conceive and only take a supplement for a single vitamin or mineral if your doctor agrees you have a special need or deficiency. If you are on a strict vegan diet, for example, you may need a vitamin B12 injection or supplement. But as a general rule you should try to get the extra nutrients you need through your diet.

Cutting down on tea and coffee

Since the first coffee houses opened in Europe in 1650, drinking a cup of tea and coffee has become an important part of any social gathering.

Coffee was first produced in Ethiopia over a thousand years ago, and people have been enjoying the stimulating effects of caffeine ever since. Coffee beans, tea leaves and cocoa beans all contain caffeine and its close relative theophylline.

Although we tend to think of these sources as harmless parts of our daily diet, these active chemicals can have a significant effect on our bodies. But does this mean that drinking too much tea, coffee, cola or even chocolate can cause damage to your health? Could they even prove to be a risk to male and female fertility?

Make no mistake, caffeine is a potent drug that is known for its stimulating properties and is also used widely in painkillers and cold remedies to enhance the effect of analgesics such as paracetamol. Caffeine-containing drinks are popular because of the lift that they give us, helping to wake us up in the morning or muster that little extra bit of energy to face an hour of work late in the day. Many people also find that caffeine helps to suppress their appetite, making dieting easier. However, it can disturb your sleep pattern, leading to permanent overtiredness, and cause withdrawal headaches if you vary your intake from day to day.

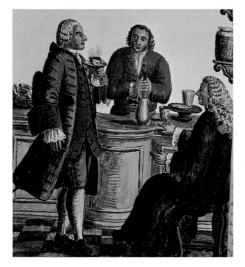

Although caffeine has never been shown to cause infertility, several research studies have suggested that drinking as little as between two and four cups of tea or coffee a day may delay conception. However, the results could be more complex than they first appear. This is because women who drink large amounts of coffee also tend to smoke. Therefore, in some cases, it could be the smoking, which is known to decrease fertility (see chapter 8:Quitting Bad Habits), that accounts for the statistics rather than a woman's high intake of caffeinated drinks.

Careful analysis of other studies of the possible effects of caffeine on the risk of miscarriage or birth defects has been reassuring as well. The weight of current scientific opinion seems to support the view that drinking tea and coffee does not significantly compromise your fertility. However, there may be other good reasons for cutting down a bit if you drink a lot of tea or coffee. Tea, for example, contains tannin, which can bind iron and stop you absorbing it; you should certainly avoid tea when you are eating an iron-rich meal. During pregnancy, you may find coffee rather nauseating – indeed, for some women this is one of the earliest signs of pregnancy. Caffeine is also more potent at this time, and will take longer to disappear from your bloodstream. So, overall, it seems sensible now that you are planning a pregnancy to cut your intake to one or two cups a day, or to switch to decaffeinated drinks or herbal or fruit teas. This will also help you get the rest you need as you prepare to conceive.

THE HEALTHY ALTERNATIVE

While you are preparing for pregnancy, why not replace tea and coffee with a fruit or herbal tea instead? As well as being caffeine-free, these teas can also be a safe and natural way to help relieve minor ailments and aid relaxation.

Some alternatives to tea and coffee include blackcurrant, blackberry, rosehip, apple, hibiscus and nettle tea. Camomile tea is good for inducing calm and sleep, and peppermint is good for indigestion. If you are suffering from a cold, squeeze half a lemon into a cup, add a spoonful of honey, a pinch of grated fresh or ground ginger and fill the cup with boiling water. To boost female fertility try drinking clover flower tea or nettle tea. For male fertility try oat and sarsaparilla tea.

Herbal remedies can relieve minor ailments such as headaches, colds or PMS. Many herbal medicines can be every bit as potent as modern drugs, however, so only take them under the supervision of a qualified herbalist who should know that you are planning to conceive. Some herbs, such as autumn crocus, aloe vera, barberry, broom, cohosh roots, feverfew, golden seal, juniper, penny royal, poke root, raspberry leaf, southern wood, tansy and thuja are dangerous during pregnancy, so avoid these as soon as you stop using contraception.

Other common herbs and spices that should be avoided in medicinal form are nutmeg and parsley, although they are safe if you use them to flavour your cooking because they are less concentrated. If you're in doubt about the safety of any herbs, spices, or fruit teas consult the manufacturer or a qualified herbalist.

Food-borne infections

Because certain foods can cause health problems that may affect a developing embryo – particularly during those vital early weeks of pregnancy – you should always take care to avoid food-borne infections in your preconception period as you prepare for pregnancy. Two of the more dangerous infections that are known to have adverse effects on your baby during pregnancy are listeriosis and toxoplasmosis. These can both be caught from food and animals but, with care, can be avoided.

Toxoplasmosis

This is caused by a parasite called Toxoplasma gondii. It is carried by many animals, found in the faeces of cats, and is also found in raw meat and unpasteurised milk. Toxoplasmosis is a common infection, but once you have had it you usually become immune to it (about 30 per cent of adults are immune). A simple blood test before pregnancy will let you know if you carry the antibodies that will protect you and your baby from toxoplasmosis.

It's important to avoid this infection while you are planning to conceive and when pregnant because treatment with antibiotics is difficult and the infection can lead to blindness and brain damage in your baby. If you know you have the antibodies, you should be safe from infection. However,

Preventing food-borne infections

To avoid listeriosis, toxoplasmosis, and other food-borne infection, follow these simple guidelines:

- Cut out liver, paté, soft cheeses, foods made with raw egg and raw or undercooked meat from your diet.
- Always keep your hands, utensils and work surfaces clean when preparing food.
- Use a separate chopping board for preparing raw meat. Plastic boards are better than wood ones because they harbour less bacteria.
- Cook raw foods thoroughly – especially meat, eggs, shellfish and pulses.
- Keep the temperature of your refrigerator below 32°F(4°C) and store raw meat on the bottom shelf to prevent juices dripping onto other foodstuffs. All foods in the fridge should also be covered.
- Use a cool bag to transport frozen foods from the store to your home.
- Always buy and eat food before the "sell by" and "use by" dates listed on the packaging.
- Always follow manufacturers' instructions when defrosting and reheating precooked foods.
- Make sure food is reheated to steaming hot for at least two minutes, and throw away any left-over reheated food.
- Do not refreeze defrosted food.
- Wash your hands after handling animals.
- Wash pet utensils separately from your own utensils.

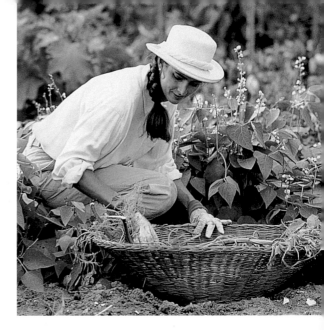

it's best to take preventative measures. You should always wash your hands each time you have handled a cat or kitten. If possible, avoid touching cat litter or use gloves and wash your hands afterwards. Always empty litter trays within 24 hours as the parasite is not active before this time. Be sure to wash vegetables carefully (especially those to be eaten raw), avoid drinking or cooking with unpasteurised milk, and cook raw meat thoroughly.

Listeriosis

This is caused by the bacteria Listeria monocytogenes. It can be found in soil and water, and is carried by some animals, such as pregnant or lambing sheep. Also found in many foods such as soft cheeses and patés, it is an unusual bacteria because it can multiply in the low temperatures found in your fridge. Heating foods to at least 70°C (160°F) for more than two minutes will kill the bacteria.

To lessen the risk of becoming infected with toxoplasmosis, wear gloves when gardening as soil can often be contaminated by cats.

A bout of listeriosis is usually very mild, rather like having the flu, and it can be treated with antibiotics. But if you are infected during pregnancy, the bacteria can cross the placenta and seriously affect your baby, even possibly causing miscarriage or stillbirth. Even though the bacteria is found widely in food, it doesn't often cause problems in pregnancy and is less common than toxoplasmosis. Despite its rarity, you should try to avoid it, especially around the time of conception and pregnancy. To reduce the risk of listeriosis, cut out soft cheeses like Brie or Camembert and blue-veined varieties. Avoid paté, which is often a carrier of the infection. You should also be very careful when eating ready-made "cook/chill" meals, reheating them thoroughly for at least two minutes so that they are steaming hot.

Body weight and your fertility

A healthy body weight is crucial for optimum fertility, but before you groan at the thought of stepping on the scales, read on. The popular image of an apparently healthy, young and slim female is far from ideal when it comes to getting pregnant. In fact, your ideal body weight for fertility is probably heavier than you think.

The female body needs to carry a certain amount of fat before the hypothalamus and pituitary glands in the brain can send out sufficient levels of hormones to stimulate the ovaries into releasing an ovum. Most young

Your diet in pregnancy

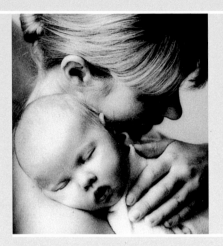

You may be surprised to learn that if you were already eating a healthy diet before you became pregnant, you probably won't need to change it very much to cover the extra nutritional demands of pregnancy. This is because your body adapts during pregnancy and becomes more efficient at absorbing some minerals, such as iron. You will also be able to utilise some stored vitamins and minerals, such as Vitamins B12 and D, and iron.

Changes to your diet

Despite the fact that your body will adapt in preparation for pregnancy, it is still important that you keep up a healthy intake of all the important vitamins and minerals (such as B12 and calcium) so that your body can replenish its stores.

Your body will demand more calories and a little more protein to cope with the growth of your baby, the placenta, your expanding breasts and uterus. The exact amount of extra energy you need will depend on how much you reduce your exercise (many women tend to conserve energy in early pregnancy because fatigue prevents them from being as active). Make sure you increase your calorie intake through starchy sources that are also rich in vitamins and minerals (for example, wholemeal bread) instead of chocolate and crisps.

You also need to steer clear of certain foods such as liver, paté, soft cheeses, foods made with raw egg, and raw or undercooked meat. These can all carry infections, which may be a risk to your baby (see page 98).

Coping with morning sickness

Nausea and vomiting in the early weeks of pregnancy can often prevent some women from getting the nutrients they require. To help reduce the problem of morning sickness (which can occur at any time of the day), there are a number of simple rules to follow from the time you

hope to conceive and certainly from the moment you know you are pregnant.

First of all, never miss a meal – hunger is a sure recipe for nausea in pregnancy. Next, avoid eating large, heavy meals and eat smaller portions more frequently instead. Eat a starchy snack, such as dry oat biscuits or rice crackers, or dried fruit every two to three hours to keep up your energy intake. Have a snack before you go to sleep and before you get out of bed every morning. Finally, avoid tea and coffee (see page 96) and don't let yourself get too tired.

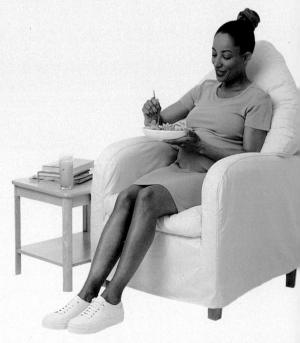

girls need to reach a weight of around 48 kg (106 lbs or 7 stone) before starting their first period, but to maintain your fertility you need to be heavier than this. In the late teenage years most women put on at least 10 kg (22 lbs or 1½ stone) as they grow taller and store body fat in all the familiar places.

Low body weight and sudden weight loss cause a temporary halt in the supply of luteinising hormone (LH) and follicle stimulating hormone (FSH) from the brain, meaning that the ovaries are not stimulated so no ovum is released (see chapter 1: The Fertile Body). This natural safety mechanism prevents babies from being conceived when the mother is short of food. Unfortunately, many women can still conceive despite being underweight. Women who start a pregnancy in these circumstances face a higher risk of miscarriage or of their baby being born underweight or prematurely. Infants with low birth weights are vulnerable to infection and prone to feeding difficulties in the first few weeks of life.

Your ideal body weight

The ideal body weight for a woman's fertility covers a wide range, but if you are at the low or high end of the range, you may start to have irregular periods, and this can decrease your fertility.

The best way to calculate your ideal body weight is to use the Body Mass Index (BMI), which appears on the following page. For the optimum chance of getting pregnant, your weight for height should give you a BMI somewhere around the mid 20s. A BMI of under 20 indicates that you are underweight and obesity is usually defined as a BMI of above 30.

If your BMI is outside the fertile range you may want to delay conception until you gain or lose weight (see the box on page 103). If your BMI is ideal but you still feel overweight, now is not the time to diet. Instead, take moderate exercise to tone up your muscles (see chapter 7: Improving Your Physical and Emotional Health) and improve the quality of your diet. If your BMI is lower than the mid 20s, read on and consider delaying conception while you adjust your diet to give your body the resources it needs. As a rule of thumb, if you let your body weight fall to a BMI less than 18 you are very likely to suffer from temporary infertility. About 50 per cent of women who have a BMI below 20 stop ovulating and have fertility problems.

If you are taking the combined oral contraceptive pill, you will probably get regular pill periods even if your body weight is low. This may give you the impression that your body weight is healthy. However, periods that you have while you are taking the pill are only artificial bleeds (see page

?

DID YOU KNOW?

Being underweight is one of the most common reasons for female infertility caused by ovulation failure. In one study at the University of Mississippi in 1982, a group of underweight women who suffered from unexplained infertility were put on an enriched diet to increase their body weight. Of these, 75 per cent went on to conceive spontaneously as their weight increased and did not need any further help from the clinic.

70), and when you stop taking the pill you may not get a period regularly until your weight is in the ideal fertile range.

The dangers of dieting

Many women believe they are overweight and that a healthy body must be a thin one. There is no doubt that obesity is a problem in Western society

The Body Mass Index (BMI) chart was designed to discover your optimum body weight. The green area indicates the ideal BMI range for a woman planning to get pregnant.

ST	PD	KG	BODY MASS INDEX																
14½	203	92	39	38	37	36	36	35	34	33	32	31	31	30	29	29	28	27	27
			39	38	37	36	35	34	33	33	32	31	30	30	29	28	28	27	27
			39	38	37	36	35	34	33	32	32	31	30	29	29	28	27	27	26
14	196	89	38	37	36	35	34	34	33	32	31	30	30	29	28	28	27	27	26
			38	37	36	35	34	33	32	32	31	30	29	29	28	27	27	26	26
			37	36	35	34	34	33	32	31	30	30	29	28	28	27	27	26	25
13½	189	86	37	36	35	34	33	32	32	31	30	29	29	28	27	27	26	26	25
			36	35	35	34	33	32	31	30	30	29	28	28	27	27	26	26	25
			36	35	34	33	32	32	31	30	29	29	28	27	27	26	26	25	25
13	182	83	35	35	34	33	32	31	30	30	29	28	28	27	26	26	25	25	24
			35	34	33	32	32	31	30	29	29	28	27	27	26	26	25	24	24
			35	34	33	32	31	30	30	29	28	28	27	26	26	25	25	24	24
12½	175	79	35	33	32	32	31	30	29	29	28	27	27	26	26	25	25	24	23
			34	33	32	31	30	30	29	28	28	27	26	26	25	25	24	24	23
			34	32	32	31	30	29	29	28	27	27	26	25	25	24	24	23	23
12	168	76	33	32	31	30	30	29	28	28	27	26	26	25	25	24	24	23	22
			33	32	31	30	29	29	28	27	27	26	25	25	24	24	23	23	22
			32	31	30	30	29	28	28	27	26	26	25	24	24	23	23	22	22
11½	161	73	32	31	30	29	29	28	27	26	26	25	25	24	24	23	23	22	22
			32	30	30	29	28	27	27	26	26	25	24	24	23	23	22	22	21
			31	30	29	28	28	27	26	26	25	25	24	23	23	22	22	21	21
11	154	70	31	30	29	28	27	27	26	25	25	24	24	23	23	22	22	21	21
			30	29	28	28	27	26	26	25	24	24	23	23	22	22	21	21	20
			30	29	28	27	27	26	26	25	24	24	23	22	22	21	21	21	20
10½	147	67	29	28	28	27	26	26	25	24	24	23	23	22	22	21	21	20	20
			29	28	27	26	26	25	25	24	23	23	22	22	21	21	20	20	19
			29	27	27	26	25	25	24	24	23	22	22	21	21	21	20	20	19
10	140	64	28	27	26	26	25	24	24	23	23	22	22	21	21	20	20	19	19
			28	27	26	25	25	24	23	23	22	22	21	21	20	20	19	19	19
			27	26	25	25	24	24	23	22	22	21	21	20	20	20	19	19	18
9½	133	60	27	26	25	24	24	23	23	22	22	21	21	20	20	19	19	18	18
			26	25	25	24	23	23	22	22	21	21	20	20	19	19	19	18	18
			26	25	24	24	23	22	22	21	21	20	20	19	19	19	18	18	17
9	126	57	26	24	24	23	23	22	22	21	21	20	20	19	19	18	18	18	17
			25	24	23	23	22	22	21	21	20	20	19	19	18	18	18	17	17
			25	24	23	22	22	21	21	20	20	19	19	18	18	18	17	17	17
8½	119	54	24	23	23	22	21	21	20	20	19	19	19	18	18	17	17	17	16
			24	23	22	22	21	21	20	20	19	19	18	18	17	17	17	16	16
			23	22	22	21	21	20	20	19	19	18	18	18	17	17	16	16	16
8	112	51	23	22	21	21	20	20	19	19	18	18	18	17	17	16	16	16	15
			23	22	21	20	20	19	19	19	18	18	17	17	16	16	15	15	15
			22	21	21	20	20	19	19	18	18	17	17	17	16	16	15	15	15
7½	105	48	22	21	20	20	19	19	18	18	17	17	17	16	16	15	15	15	14
			21	20	20	19	19	18	18	17	17	17	16	16	15	15	15	14	14
			20	20	19	19	18	18	17	17	17	16	16	15	15	15	14	14	14
7	98	45	20	19	19	18	18	18	17	17	16	16	16	15	15	15	14	14	14
			19	19	18	18	18	17	17	16	16	16	15	15	15	14	14	14	13
			19	19	18	18	17	17	16	16	16	15	15	15	14	14	14	13	13
6½	91	41	19	18	18	17	17	16	16	16	15	15	15	14	14	14	13	13	13
			18	18	17	17	16	16	16	15	15	15	14	14	14	13	13	13	12
			18	17	17	16	16	16	15	15	15	14	14	14	13	13	13	12	12
			17	17	16	16	16	15	15	15	14	14	14	13	13	13	12	12	12
METERS			1.52		1.56		1.6		1.64		1.68		1.72		1.76		1.80		1.84
INCHES			5'0	5'1	5'2	5'3	5'4	5'5	5'6	5'7	5'8	5'9	5'10	5'11	6'0				

and, combined with little exercise, can increase the risk of health problems. However, women who lose weight unnecessarily may jeopardise their chances of becoming pregnant and having a healthy baby. Dieting for weight loss is much the same to your body as starvation and can lead to ovulation failure and a disturbed menstrual cycle. Even if you are overweight, rapid weight loss can disturb your menstrual cycle and a drastic reduction in what you eat will cause shortages of many vital nutrients, many of which the body cannot store and are needed every day (vitamin C, for example). For safe weight loss, see the box below.

Male fertility and body weight

Low body weight is not such a common cause of male infertility, but severe weight loss through illness or anorexia can reduce the quantity and quality of a man's sperm count. Obesity can decrease testosterone production and can also depress a man's libido. If your partner is overweight, perhaps the prospect of fatherhood will give him the motivation he needs to lose some weight by improving his diet and increasing the amount of exercise he does.

Losing and gaining weight safely

To lose weight try the following:

- Don't lose more than 2 lbs a week. A slow and steady approach will have longer-lasting effects. Only aim to get into the ideal weight range, not at the bottom of it!
- Reduce your calorie intake by limiting your fat consumption, especially animal and dairy fats, but keep your iron and calcium intake up.
- Include more fresh fruits, vegetables and skimmed dairy products in your diet.
- Do more exercise so that you can eat plenty of nutrient-rich food but still lose weight.
- Discuss your form of contraception with your doctor if you feel it is affecting your weight.

To gain weight, try the following:

- Consume plenty of starchy foods, vegetables and fish rich in oils.
- Eat according to your appetite, and always have regular meals.
- Even though you may be tempted to reach for biscuits and sweets in order to bump up your calorie intake, try to resist these foods as they fill you up and will prevent you from eating the more nutritious foods that your body needs.

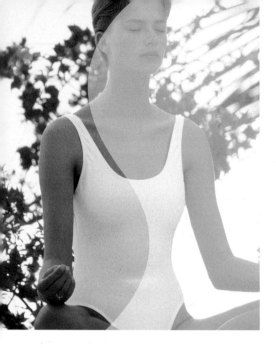

Improving Your Physical and Emotional Health

Exercising regularly and being emotionally well will bring major benefits during your preconception period and beyond. Increased fitness raises your libido (an obvious bonus when you plan to conceive!) and helps you to cope with the physical demands of pregnancy. What's more, when you are in good emotional health you are more likely to be fully fertile and conceive easily.

Physical fitness and reproductive health

You do not have to be physically fit to be fertile, but keeping yourself in good shape will improve your chances of conceiving easily and help you to have a healthy pregnancy and birth. Regular, moderate exercise reduces stress levels, promotes relaxation, and improves both mental and physical well-being. Along with a good diet, this will help you to achieve the ideal conditions for conception and pregnancy.

The benefits of exercise

Regular, moderate exercise enhances your health by generally improving both your mood and your physical well-being. Exercise gives you strength and stamina, promotes natural relaxation and encourages satisfying sleep patterns. It also increases the heart's capacity to pump efficiently and keeps blood pressure low: small blood vessels open up in the exercised muscles, reducing resistance to blood flow. This not only helps to prevent heart disease in the long-term, but also helps during pregnancy when your heart has to work harder than usual to deliver blood to the growing placenta and your own expanding body.

More specifically, regular, moderate exercise can improve your fertility. It is a great way to beat stress, raise your energy levels and boost your confidence and self-esteem – all of which do wonders for your sex drive! This is one of the reasons why a sport you enjoy can play such a vital role in the preconception period. Exercising regularly also improves the blood supply to your reproductive organs and helps you prepare your body for pregnancy and labour. What's more, moderate exercise can regulate your menstrual cycle by helping you reach a healthy body weight, maintain a balanced diet and reduce the effects of anxiety. For men, exercise helps to enhance their fertility by increasing blood supply to the testes, improving libido and keeping body weight in the healthy range.

Exercise also allows you to increase your vitamin and mineral intake naturally – and improve your diet by eating more – without putting on weight. If you get little daily exercise you need only a low-energy diet because you don't eat as much, and you don't eat a wide variety of foods to provide you with all the vitamins and minerals you need. In any case, many nutrients are needed in steady amounts regardless of your calorie intake. Women need enough iron, for instance, to replace iron lost during menstruation. Walking three miles, for example, will burn up about 300 calories – the equivalent of three slices of wholegrain bread containing one quarter of your daily iron requirements.

Since obesity can prevent women from ovulating, keeping fit is also beneficial because it can help you lose weight (see also page 103). This was illustrated by the results of a study of overweight women suffering from anovulatory infertility, conducted in 1995 by the University of Adelaide in Australia. After a six-month programme of diet and exercise, where the average weight loss was about 6.3 kilograms (14 pounds or 1 stone), 12 out of 13 women started ovulating again and 11 of these became pregnant.

Even if you exercise for as little as 20 minutes, you will feel a sense of general well-being and relaxation afterwards. This effect is not just due to the sense of achievement you feel or because it was fun; there is also a biochemical basis. When you exercise, chemicals called endorphins are released into your circulation. Similar to morphine, endorphins are the body's natural opiates and have a positive effect on the brain (see box on page 106).

The benefits of keeping fit are most noticeable when you exercise consistently. Sudden, vigorous bursts of exercise after weeks of inactivity will only wear you out. A thirty-minute session of moderate exercise, taken regularly and within your own personal fitness limits, is much better.

Working exercise into your life

The amount of exercise you need to include in your life depends on how active you are already. Obviously, if you spend all day in an office environment you will need to build in more exercise than if you have a physically demanding job as a nurse, for example.

Experts generally agree that you need a minimum of three 20–30 minute sessions of exercise a week to keep your body healthy. Even this amount, though, is very little compared to the amount of physical activity

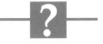

DID YOU KNOW?

A study in 1996 conducted by Dr Roger Miensset at the University of Toulouse in France showed that couples experienced up to six months' delay in conceiving if the male partner's job involved driving for more than three hours a day. As well as the negative effects of insufficient exercise, sitting in a car for long hours with poor ventilation keeps the testes too warm, and this can lower a man's sperm count. So much for the car being a symbol of male virility!

ENDORPHINS: THE FEEL GOOD FACTOR

Why is it that you feel so elated after half an hour in the gym, despite the sweat running down your back and the hair plastered all over your face? The answer lies in the various physiological changes that occur in the body when you work out.

When you exercise, the blood flow throughout your body increases, making you feel warm and relaxed. This effect can also be seen by changes in electrical activity in the brain: the alpha waves – generally associated with a relaxed mind – increase. Exercising also helps to relieve stress by allowing a physical outlet for all the tension and stress that can build up in your muscles from day to day.

Another major factor contributing to your sense of well-being after exercise is the release of endorphins. Released by the pituitary gland in the brain, endorphins are opiates and have a similar chemical effect on the body to morphine, blocking pain and promoting a state of euphoria. Like morphine, endorphins (which are also responsible for the natural high experienced during orgasm) can be addictive. This may help to explain why some people become so hooked on sports.

The powerful effect of endorphins was demonstrated by an experiment conducted in 1992 by a Canadian, Dr Daniel, on a group of volunteers who had been doing regular aerobics for six months. Half the group were given an endorphin-blocking drug before an aerobics session, while the others were given an inactive injection. Neither group was aware which of the two injections they had been given. After the exercise session, the group who had not been given the active drug generally felt better and reported feelings of calmness, reduced anger, tension, and fatigue. However, the group whose endorphins had been inhibited by the drug noticed no such improvement in their mood.

Endorphins are released in vast quantities during childbirth as well as during exercise. Acting at various sites in the brain, spinal cord and at the nervous endings, endorphins help to block the pain of childbirth naturally.

that was an essential part of everyday life only a few decades ago. Many common health problems today, including obesity and osteoporosis, are closely related to lack of exercise. Cars, washing machines, food processors and hundreds of other labour-saving devices have deprived us of the daily activities that once kept us much fitter. Generally we need far more exercise than modern living provides, and this means that we need to build more physical activity into our lives.

If you know you are out of condition, start by improving your suppleness with gentle exercise, such as swimming, walking, low impact aerobics, or relaxation exercises, once or twice a week. Once you feel in better shape, increase your stamina by making these exercise sessions more frequent and adding in some more vigorous exercise, such as jogging, aerobics, racket sports or cycling. Any activity that makes you sweat a little, get slightly out of breath, and causes your pulse rate to rise (see page 109) is good for building up your fitness. You should be able to carry on exercising for 20 minutes but still have enough breath to talk as you go.

Try also to keep supple by incorporating plenty of stretching into your everyday body movements – both in your leisure time and at work. With a bit of thought, even mundane household chores can be transformed into useful exercises. For example, stretching your arms to hang the laundry out rather than using the tumble dryer, or scrubbing the kitchen floor on all fours rather than using a mop will help you to stretch and use your whole body. Taking the stairs instead of the lift and walking instead of driving will also give a significant boost to your weekly physical activities. Leisure activities such as gardening, dancing, and even strolling in the park with the dog are all ways to incorporate more exercise into your life.

Looking ahead to pregnancy, it's a good idea to get into the habit of squatting if you want to pick something up or talk to a small child, rather than bending over. This will help to improve the suppleness and strength of your pelvic floor area and protect your back from any possible strain. For more information on exercising during pregnancy, turn to page 110.

You can increase the amount of exercise you do as much as you like, so long as your body weight remains in the fertile range (see page 101) and your menstrual cycle stays regular. Exercising should be fun rather than punishing, so try to choose something you enjoy doing. Exercising with a friend is another way to increase the fun factor, as well as give yourself motivation and hold you to your plans.

Can too much exercise affect your fertility?

Frequent, vigorous exercise and physical training for sports such as marathon running, ballet and gymnastics can affect your ability to conceive. Young girls who train hard for these sports, particularly if their body weight is low, often experience a delay in the onset of menstruation. Older women who practice endurance training, in which they continually exercise to their physical limits, may also begin to miss periods or even stop menstruating altogether. Up to 50 per cent of women athletes report irregular or absent periods. Running more than 20 miles a week may delay conception by causing irregular ovulation, as may vigorous training for more than an hour or so each day.

A demanding exercise regime is more likely to inhibit ovulation if your body fat stores are low. Because oestrogen levels fall when the body's fat stores are depleted, scientists believe that this, in turn, prevents the pituitary gland in the brain from releasing the surge of luteinising hormone required to trigger ovulation. Some women athletes, such as swimmers,

SPORTS TO HELP YOU GET FIT

Each sport benefits your health in slightly different ways. For example, while jogging can be great for improving stamina and burning calories, swimming will do more for your flexibility. Some sports are safe in the preconception period but are not suitable for pregnancy, (see Looking Ahead on page 110). Safe exercise should improve your stamina and suppleness but not have a risk of injury in pregnancy. The chart below rates the virtues of each exercise per 20-minute session and indicates whether it is safe to pursue in pregnancy. Remember to warm up beforehand and wind down gradually.

ACTIVITY	CALORIES USED	STAMINA	SUPPLENESS	SAFE IN PREGNANCY
Aerobics	150	•••	•••	If within fitness limits
Basketball	110	••	••	If within fitness limits
Cycling	100-150	••	•	Yes
Dancing (ballroom)	100	••	•	Yes
(disco/club)	150	••	•	Yes
Decorating/housework	70	•	••	Yes
Golf	90	••	•	Yes
Gymnastics	120	•••	•••	If within fitness limits
Horse riding (gentle hacking)	70	•	••	Yes
(jumping)	90	••	••	No
Jogging	120	•••	••	Yes
Martial arts (kickboxing/judo)	90	••	••	No
Netball	110	••	••	If within fitness limits
Racket sports	100	••	••	Yes
Rock climbing	90	••	••	No
Sailing	80	•	••	Yes
Scuba diving	110	••	••	No
Skiing downhill	100	••	••	No
Skipping	150	•••	••	Yes
Sprint running	150	•••	••	If within fitness limits
Swimming	130	•••	•••	Yes
Walking (in town)	80	•	•	Yes
(hill walking)	150	•••	••	If within fitness limits
Waterskiing	100	••	••	No
Weight training	100	••	••	If within fitness limits
Yoga	40	•	••	Yes

tend to maintain a normal body weight because of their high muscle bulk, yet they can still find it difficult to conceive because their fat stores are low and their periods are irregular due to low oestrogen levels.

It may seem strange that very fit women should be less fertile than others, but once a woman athlete does conceive the outlook for her pregnancy is just as good. The key for any woman wanting to keep up regular sports and plan for a pregnancy is to eat enough to maintain a healthy body weight and to monitor her menstrual cycle to ensure it remains fairly regular. If your periods are infrequent, learning fertility awareness (see chapter 3) will help you to determine your most fertile times.

Exercise for men While endurance training seems less likely to affect fertility in men than it does in women, it can still have a profound effect on a man's sperm count. Long-distance running has been shown to inhibit testosterone levels and reduce sperm count, which could be a problem for men who started with a low sperm count for another reason. Because the

How fit are you?

Before you exercise, test your overall fitness to ensure you work out at the appropriate level of intensity. Most health clubs employ trained fitness experts who will take into account your personal endurance, strength, stamina, lifestyle and medical health to provide a thorough assessment of your physical condition.

You can test your general fitness yourself. A simple way is to see if you can walk briskly for 15 minutes without getting out of breath. Another way is to take your resting pulse rate first thing in the morning. Find your pulse on the side of your neck underneath your jawbone or on the inside of your wrist. Use your forefinger or middle finger and press down gently, but firmly on to the pulse.

Once you can feel your pulse, count the number of beats over a 15-second period, then multiply this by four to get your resting pulse rate. If it is under 70 you are in good condition. If it's between 80 and 100 you are a little out of shape. A resting pulse of 100 or more indicates you are in poor physical health. Remember that anxiety (see page 115) also raises your pulse.

Regular exercise lowers your resting pulse rate by making your heart more efficient (some athletes have resting pulses as low as 40). It also reduces the time it takes for your pulse to return to normal after exercising.

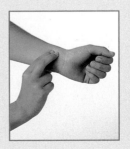
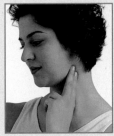

Exercise during pregnancy

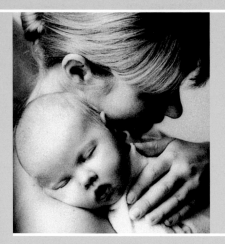

Most sports are safe to pursue in pregnancy. If you were already fit, exercising while pregnant won't decrease the blood supply to your baby's placenta. Because your body temperature is higher in pregnancy, wear loose clothing and drink plenty of water to avoid becoming overheated. You may also tire more easily than before, so stop as soon as you feel tired or breathless, especially as your baby gets bigger.

Sports that are safe

Swimming is an ideal sport when you are pregnant because it keeps your body well supported, especially the joints (when you are pregnant, the hormone progesterone has a softening effect on the ligaments surrounding your joints, which makes them vulnerable to damage). Cycling and other non-weight bearing activities are also good sports to pursue while you are pregnant.

Sports to avoid

Some water sports, such as waterskiing, should be avoided during pregnancy because they carry a risk of the vagina being douched with water under pressure, causing infection or damage to the protective membranes surrounding your baby. Scuba diving at all stages of pregnancy should be avoided because the equipment required can restrict your circulation and the decompression you experience may affect your baby.

From the second trimester avoid all high-impact sports, such as skiing and horseback riding. If you fall they could cause serious injury and, in theory, disrupt the attachment of the placenta. Many top-class athletes continue training throughout pregnancy, but marathon running and prolonged aerobics at endurance level raise your core body temperature and can decrease the placenta's blood flow to your baby. Sweating cools you off, but it does not let your uterus cool down, so while you might feel better, your baby is hot!

Exercising on your back (as is common in aerobics) can affect your circulation and cause dizziness from the fifth month, as well as cause stomach muscle strain. Avoid positions that cause your uterus to press directly on the blood vessels lying along your spine, and lie on your side instead. Try to find an exercise class designed especially for pregnant mothers.

Although you can continue exercising until the end of your pregnancy, most experts recommend tapering off in the last few weeks. Stretching, swimming and walking should provide adequate exercise and keep you supple.

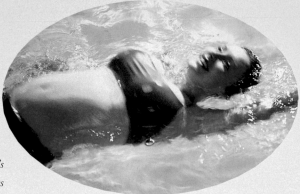

testes hang outside the body, the raised body temperature which results from exercise usually does not affect a man's fertility. Nevertheless, men should avoid overheating by wearing loose clothing and cooling off afterwards, perhaps with a shower.

While good physical health – including a healthy diet and avoiding such hazards as smoking, drugs and irradiation – is vital to successful conception and pregnancy, so too is your emotional state. Although it is quite possible to conceive in a state of great psychological turmoil, you are more likely to be fully fertile when you are emotionally healthy. Our bodies have remarkable inbuilt mechanisms which help to prevent us from conceiving when we are not ready for it. In chapter 6 we saw how we are less likely to ovulate when our bodies sense food supplies are short, and in a similar way, the hypothalamus can switch off its supply of stimulating hormones when it senses we are under extreme emotional stress or pressure.

Emotional fitness and reproductive health

What is good emotional health?

Most people can recognise in either themselves or others signs of emotional strain in moments of anxiety, perhaps over a job interview, during the stress of moving house, or in times of grief or bereavement. But good emotional health can be a harder concept to pin down.

Although it may seem obvious, it is healthy to experience a variety of emotions, including joy, sadness, anger, fear, pleasure, interest, boredom, anxiety, boldness, guilt or pride. In fact, you need a complete range of emotions to experience life to the full and to give vital feedback in relationships. One of the early signs of depression, for instance, is a blunting of all feelings.

Another hallmark of good emotional health is the ability to respond to your feelings at appropriate times, facing them rather than fearing them. Some reactions, such as pleasure, are easy to understand and pass quickly. But anger or disappointment over an apparently trivial incident can be puzzling or even shocking. Your reactions to events can provide insights into aspects of your emotional well-being that would otherwise stay hidden. This is not advice to become unhealthily introspective but a reminder that good emotional health includes facing ourselves as we are, and being prepared to adapt or change.

Nobody knows what the future holds for them, but a sign of good emotional health is being able to plan ahead without feeling stressed. As well as looking forwards, you should also be able to face your past, which

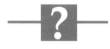

DID YOU KNOW?

Out of nearly 2,000 couples investigated for infertility by the Women's Hospital of the Free University of Berlin Charlottenburg in 1988, approximately 25 per cent were found to have a psychological cause for their infertility. Although other figures worldwide may not always be this high, emotional fitness and a healthy relationship can be crucial for your fertility.

can be harder. Of course you cannot change the past, but you can change the way you think about it. Being prepared to deal with any pain or anxieties that still plague you can be of enormous benefit in improving your mental well-being. Although the past might seem irrelevant, you may be surprised at how much your physical health, and even your fertility, can improve when you begin to feel more at peace with yourself.

Some people love company and others can happily spend hours alone, but anyone in good emotional health should be able to face either prospect without a problem. Dreading meeting people or the opposite, that you cannot bear to be on your own, may be a symptom of an inner fear or turmoil that is likely to be putting you under stress.

Some aspects of physical health can reflect a person's emotional state. Who hasn't experienced a sleepless night worrying about an event the next day or suddenly lost their appetite when they heard some bad news? These short-lived changes in the body's habits are normal reactions to stressful events but, when emotionally healthy, you should recover quickly and be able to see the cause of the problem. Eating and sleeping properly, as well as being able to relax, are signs of being in good emotional health.

Finally, when you are emotionally well, your relationships with other people should be healthy. If you find your relationships are suddenly becoming strained, it may be a sign that your own emotional state is upset, rather than there being a problem with the relationship itself.

What is stress?

Stress is any force that places physical or emotional demands on us. Some people think of stress as an entirely negative influence, but for others it is the goad they need to achieve their ambitions. Any challenging experience is, to some extent, stressful – whether it is something as mundane as meeting the daily deadline to get to work on time, or a major event such as moving house or a bereavement. Even happy events like marriage, having a baby, or winning the lottery can be surprisingly stressful.

The common factor in all these potentially stressful situations is the element of change. Change has to be stressful or you could not adapt to it. In fact, like it or not, some stress is vital to a healthy lifestyle! Small amounts of stress or everyday challenges can be stimulating and help to keep you alert and interested. It only becomes a problem when it acts in a negative way, making you feel pressurised and out of control. Because the hypothalamus is central to the body's response to stress (as well as your fertility) it is not surprising that prolonged stress can have a devastating effect on your fertility and sexual life.

How stress affects female fertility

By interfering with the action of the hypothalamus, severe stress can upset the normal cycle of hormones from the pituitary and disturb or inhibit ovulation, leading to irregular periods. In 1986 Dr Harrison and his colleagues at the University of Dublin, Ireland studied a group of women with unexplained infertility. They all had high levels of prolactin, a hormone associated with stress, which can also prevent ovulation. When these women were taught to relax, their prolactin levels decreased and their menstrual cycles gradually returned to normal.

FIGHT OR FLIGHT: THE STRESS RESPONSE

When you register a sudden stress or threat, your brain shuts down some of the body's systems so that all available energy can be directed towards confronting the threat or escaping from it. This is known as the "fight or flight" response – your heart beats faster, your breathing becomes quick and shallow, and blood flows away from the non-essential organs, such as the skin and stomach, and rushes instead to the muscles and brain. You may also sweat more, your mouth goes dry (less saliva is produced), and you feel the sudden urge to urinate. These effects are all brought on by the hormone adrenaline, which is released by the two adrenal glands under instructions from the hypothalamus gland in the brain.

Unfortunately, few challenges in the modern world require such a physical response, so stress can make you feel anxious without ever having a physical release. The human body can weather short bursts of stress, so long as it relaxes fully in between. But people often endure prolonged stress, and this can damage their health.

If you are under constant pressure you may suffer from minor symptoms such as irritability, muscle ache, fatigue and disturbed appetite. If you're susceptible to herpes or cystitis, you may find that stress sets off an attack. Long-term stress can lead to disturbed sleep patterns, anxiety, panic attacks, stomach ulcers, high blood pressure and chronic headaches. It can also depress your immune system, and you may find yourself catching every cough and cold around.

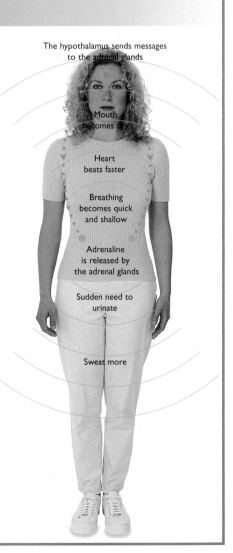

The hypothalamus sends messages to the adrenal glands

Mouth becomes dry

Heart beats faster

Breathing becomes quick and shallow

Adrenaline is released by the adrenal glands

Sudden need to urinate

Sweat more

Women's bodies vary in their sensitivity to stress, however. The prospect of a driving test might be enough to stop one woman's periods, while another may menstruate exactly on time even after the death of a close friend. Even if your periods do not stop altogether, they may become painless, light or irregular, with very short or long gaps between them. A prolonged disturbance in your menstrual cycle may be a sign that your body is rebelling against the pressure you are under. It is not unusual to hear of women who have suffered infertility for many years and been under severe stress and pressure, to conceive when that pressure was lifted. For instance, when they were accepted by an adoption agency to become adoptive parents (see case study on page 117) or given a date to start fertility treatment.

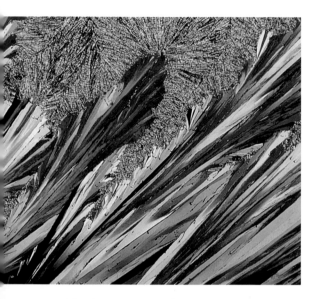

If you are under stress you may also find that you lose interest in sex and find it hard to become sexually aroused and achieve an orgasm. Just as fear can give you a dry mouth, the adrenaline released during the stress response can cause vaginal dryness by inhibiting the function of the cervical and vaginal mucus glands. If ovulation ceases in the long term, the low levels of oestrogen might reduce the ability of your vagina to respond sexually and lessen the fertile properties of cervical mucus.

Testosterone (a light micrograph of its crystals is shown above) is the hormone responsible for maintaining libido in men and, combined with oestrogen, libido in women. Testosterone levels can be affected by stress.

How stress affects male fertility

A man under stress, particularly a tired man, is likely to begin losing interest in sex. He may not enjoy making love as much as he used to and find it difficult to maintain an erection long enough to ejaculate or satisfy his partner. Stress can also cause premature ejaculation. These problems are temporary and should be relieved when the stress-related problems are resolved. (Impotence and erectile difficulties can have many causes apart from stress and this is discussed more fully in chapter 11.)

Long-term stress can also affect sperm production by interfering with the hormones from the pituitary gland that stimulate the testes. Research has shown that men under stress at work or at home are more likely to have poor sperm quality and may experience lower fertility. Stress can add to the effects of other causes of poor sperm production, such as smoking or obesity.

Anxiety and fertility

Like prolonged stress, anxiety can reduce your fertility and affect your libido. Feelings of anxiety are very similar to fear but are less severe and are quite normal in many situations. It only becomes unhealthy when you begin to feel anxious for no apparent reason or when it is out of all proportion to the cause of your worry. Symptoms of abnormal anxiety include constantly worrying about something; having the physical feelings of fear (racing pulse, sweating, goose bumps, breathlessness) without any obvious reason; difficulty sleeping; nightmares; poor concentration and memory; panic attacks about situations you could once have faced without problem (for example, supermarket shopping); prolonged muscle tension and headaches; and nausea, poor appetite or diarrhoea.

Abnormal anxiety can be caused by the suppressed emotions of a traumatic experience in the past. Childhood abuse, rape, or the loss of a baby through abortion or miscarriage can all be triggers, as can many less extreme events. Past relationships also set the stage for anxiety. Children of demanding or anxious parents often grow up to be nervous and find it hard to relax. They may set themselves impossible standards so that they constantly feel anxious to succeed. Personality has a part to play as well – some of us are just more prone to anxiety than others.

If you are severely affected by anxiety, your doctor may be able to help unravel the cause. It could be brought on by physical illness, such as an overactive thyroid (see page 171) or high blood pressure (see page 159), which not only needs treatment but could also be affecting your fertility. Be sure to mention that you are considering pregnancy if the question of medication arises. Tranquillisers (including sleeping pills) are now known to be addictive and doctors will usually prescribe them in short courses only to help people over a sudden traumatic event.

Managing stress and anxiety

If you cannot avoid stress, you can at least learn to

TIME TO TALK

Facing up to stress

Pregnancy and parenthood are major life events that will inevitably bring some measure of stress to your lives. Before you embark on a pregnancy, consider the pressures you are under and, if possible, allow yourselves the space and time to resolve – or at least confront – problems you may have. For example, you may be worried over the permanence of your marriage or relationship. Other stresses include conflict between your desire for children and your desire to pursue a career; guilt or fear surrounding a previous termination of pregnancy; unresolved grief over a previous miscarriage or stillbirth; and fear of experiencing a traumatic childbirth or postpartum depression after the birth.

Rather than resolving conflict, a new baby will make demands on your relationship and you will be glad you took the time to consider some of the emotional impact of becoming a parent before you have small children to care for.

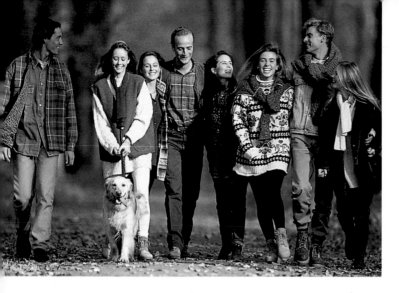

Take time out from your busy schedule to have some fun and relax with friends. Simly enjoying yourself will help to balance the stress in your life.

control its effects. In fact, you will have already taken an important step towards recovery just by recognising that you are suffering from stress or anxiety. Try listing all the worries you have, writing them down in order of severity, then work down the list and attempt to find a solution for each problem. Just sharing your worries can also be a help, so talk to your partner, a trusted friend, or a counsellor recommended by your doctor. You can also help to prevent stress and anxiety by understanding why you react as you do in certain situations and by learning a relaxation technique (see page 121).

Time management One of the best ways to beat stress is to plan ahead. You'll be surprised at how much easier it is to get everything done simply by managing your life. Start by listing everything you need to do each week. Be critical, though, and leave out anything that is unnecessary. Next, write down everything you would like to do. Include some exercise and something relaxing that you enjoy doing. Now plan a timetable for your week. Be realistic about how long each task will take, then work in a bit more time than you think you may need for each task. Organise each day so you can perform the more demanding tasks when you are most alert. Don't give the unrewarding tasks prime time. Instead, fit them into the odd moments and give priority to the things you really want to do. Time spent travelling or waiting can be used to tackle small jobs or practice relaxation. By examining and reorganising your week you can relieve anxiety by feeling more in control of your life.

If it really seems impossible to fit everything in, you may have some tough decisions to make. But letting go is more important than subjecting yourself to unreasonable stress, which can affect your health and fertility.

Depression and fertility

It is estimated that 10 per cent of men and 20 per cent of women experience depression at some time during their lives, and two out of three sufferers will lose interest in sex. Depressed women suffer from low libido and often find low sexual arousal a problem. Depressed men experience erection problems, premature ejaculation, or difficulties with orgasm.

Depression may also reduce fertility in women by acting on the hypothalamus to inhibit ovulation.

In the early stages, depression can be harder to notice than anxiety. If you have never been depressed, you may wonder how it feels. The answer is that you may feel nothing at all. It can make you aware of a deep unhappiness or stop you feeling much pain or pleasure. You forget how to laugh, lose your appetite or overeat, and your emotions seem numbed. You may feel very tired but find it impossible to sleep or, alternatively, sleep too much. The future seems bleak and everyday tasks can seem too much of an effort. Severe depression can make you feel guilty, worthless, or even so hopeless that suicide seems the only way out.

If you experience any of these symptoms you should seek medical help. Your doctor may suggest counselling and, possibly, medication. Be sure to use contraception if antidepressants are prescribed, as some antidepressants can harm a developing baby. Antidepressants can also decrease your libido; about 40 per cent of men taking antidepressants have difficulties with sex drive, impotence and ejaculation. If you choose to try one of the complementary therapies discussed below make sure you involve your

Reduced stress encourages conception

Susan and Bill already had a little boy, two-year-old Matthew, and were keen to add to their family. Unfortunately, after two years of trying, Susan still couldn't conceive.

"I had been brought up in a large family and was keen for Matthew to experience the joys of having many brothers and sisters. When Bill and I first went to our doctor to discuss not being able to get pregnant again, we had some tests, which showed that there was nothing medically wrong with us. We were both in good physical and mental health and were told to keep on trying.

After another year of trying and still no baby, we lost all hope of being able to conceive again. I couldn't bear the thought of infertility treatment so, after a great deal of discussion, Bill and I put ourselves for-

wards as adoptive parents. Meanwhile, Bill kept himself busy with his career and I distracted myself with plenty of hobbies.

Eventually we were accepted by an adoption society who said a little girl would be available to us within a year. To celebrate, we arranged a holiday. When we returned, we were told that a girl was ready to adopt. We were overwhelmed with excitement at the arrival of Ruth, and I hardly noticed that I missed my period. But when I started to feel sick a few weeks later, I took a pregnancy test and, to my amazement, it confirmed that I was pregnant! The relief at Ruth's arrival probably helped me conceive! Eight months later I gave birth to Ella, a much-loved sister for both Matthew and Ruth."

doctor if you continue to receive medical help as well. Above all, remember to allow yourself time to recover from depression before taking on the stresses of conception, pregnancy and childbirth.

Overcoming depression with counselling

Rather than giving you clear directions as to what you should do, counselling offers you the emotional space and guidance to help yourself by allowing you to explore your own thoughts, behaviours and reactions. For counselling to be truly effective, however, it's important that you find someone with whom you feel comfortable.

There are many forms of therapy and many different organisations that offer support, practical advice and counselling. Doctors' practices, places of worship and charities, for example, often have trained counsellors available who can provide emotional support and advice on relaxation and meditation. (For counselling relating to fertility problems turn to page 183.) Some people prefer to join a self-help group, where individuals help each other through their problems by discussing their feelings together. This is done with or without the help of a trained therapist. Your doctor may be able to help put you in touch with a suitable group.

A good counsellor enables you to talk through and understand your problems.

Overcoming depression with complementary therapies

Rather than taking antidepressants to treat depression, you may prefer to try a complementary therapy. There is a tremendous range of complementary therapies to choose from and all are designed to help combat the causes of stress and rebalance the body as a whole, rather than just treat the symptoms. If you are thinking of conceiving, some therapies are more suitable than others. Many herbs and aromatherapy oils, for example, should be avoided before and after you conceive (see page 97). The therapies that are listed on the following pages are safe during the preconception period in the hands of a qualified therapist.

The time you spend on your own with an alternative practitioner is often therapeutic in itself and your therapist may even take on a counselling role if your problems are stress-related. It's probably also wise to use suitable contraception while receiving treatment until you feel ready to conceive.

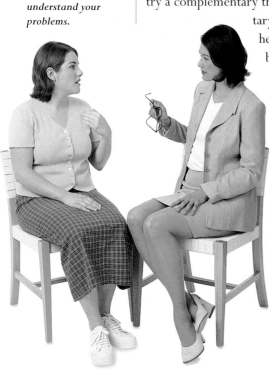

Postnatal depression

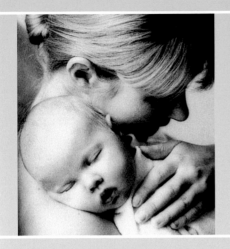

Unique to mothers of newborn babies, this affects up to one in ten first-time mothers to some degree. It's a particularly devastating illness as it comes at a time when a woman is physically vulnerable and everyone around her expects her to be happy.

A mother with postnatal depression feels very tired, despondent and unable to cope with even the simplest of tasks concerning the care of her baby. She may feel very unhappy, very guilty, inadequate and cry easily. Some mothers experience symptoms of anxiety and fear, particularly about their baby's health and may even feel pain and tension themselves. Unfortunately, as many as seven out of ten mothers who have already suffered from the illness will be affected in a subsequent pregnancy, but, with help, they can prevent it from being too serious a problem.

If you have previously suffered from postnatal depression, you may be justifiably afraid of suffering from it again and you will probably benefit from a counsellor's or therapist's support before and during your next pregnancy. Make sure you plan extra support for you and your family during the weeks after the birth. If you do develop depression, try to ask for help before it gets too severe. Your partner may be able to help you recognise the early signs. Two forms of treatment are currently being investigated to prevent the recurrence of postnatal depression. The first is to take antidepressants from late pregnancy onward, but the effects on the baby are not fully researched and will vary from one drug to another. The second is still experimental and involves the mother having high doses of progesterone by injection or pessary after the birth. Various organisations offer support to mothers with postnatal depression (see Useful Addresses on page 187), and will be able to advise you on the best course of action.

Homeopathy The principle behind homeopathic medicine is to encourage the body to heal itself. Homeopathic medicines are extremely dilute preparations of substances known to produce the symptoms they are supposed to treat – "like curing like" being the theory. They seem to be most successful at treating conditions such as allergies, skin complaints and insomnia. Many of these problems can be related to the powerful and negative effects of stress and believing that homeopathy is an effective remedy may also play a vital role in its efficacy. Always consult a qualified therapist and, as with any medicine, only take these substances on medical advice if

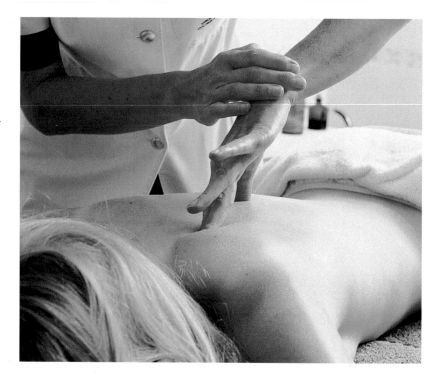

The combination of oils and massage in an aromatherapy session helps to relieve stress and nervous exhaustion.

you think you might already be pregnant (even though, by chemical standards, homeopathic medicines are so weak they are not likely to be toxic).

Aromatherapy This therapy involves massaging the body with essential plant oils. It can be an effective therapy for treating stress and nervous exhaustion because the oils both soothe and invigorate the nervous system. There are many oils you can use but always consult a trained aromatherapist before buying oils and treating yourself. A trained therapist will be able to advise you on which oils are safe and which to avoid, especially when you are trying to conceive. Aromatherapy is not recommended during the first trimester of pregnancy and many oils derived from certain herbs and plants must be avoided altogether throughout pregnancy (see page 97). Essential oils are also very concentrated, so make sure you dilute them in a carrier oil if you are going to apply them directly to the skin.

Acupuncture Practitioners of this therapy believe good health depends on the proper movement of energy, known as qi or chi, along the body's invisible energy pathways or meridians. Under stress or during emotional illness, this energy fails to flow as it should – flowing too quickly or slowly, or building up in one area at the expense of another. To restore the balance of energy in the body, acupuncturists insert very fine needles into key points along the body's meridians to release blockages and regulate the flow of energy.

Although acupuncture still defies full explanation in modern medical terms, research has shown that endorphins are released during treatment. These powerful hormones produce feelings of relaxation and well-being (see box on page 106), which may explain why acupuncture can be helpful in treating stress-related illness. Many doctors, especially pain experts, and midwives use acupuncture to relieve pain and stress in pregnant women.

Research suggests that acupuncture can be as effective as drugs in treating some infertile women who do not ovulate as a result of stress. For example, in 1992 Dr Gerhard at the University of Heidelberg, Germany, studied two groups of 45 women suffering from infrequent menstrual cycles and poor ovarian function. One group was treated with hormones and 20 out of the 45 women in that group became pregnant. The other group was treated with acupuncture and 22 women in that group became pregnant. Many of the women treated with hormones also suffered side effects but none of the women in the acupuncture group did.

Reflexology Reflexologists believe the body can be treated through the massage of specific areas on the feet or (less commonly) the hands. Each part of the body is believed to have a corresponding area on the sole of the foot or palm of the hand. While the ball of the foot is associated with the thyroid, for example, certain areas of the instep are related to the spine and liver. If an area of the foot feels sensitive or painful to touch, therapists believe that the organ to which it is connected may be weak. Massage of the appropriate foot region is then used to strengthen the affected organ.

Reflexology is thought to be helpful in treating minor ailments such as migraine, sinusitis and stress. However, practitioners of this therapy acknowledge that patients with a physical disorder should seek convention-al medical help as well. There is no reason why someone taking orthodox medicines, however, should not have sessions with a reflexologist as well.

Relaxation is a great way to enhance your physical and emotional health and, in this way, may give a general boost your fertility. When you are relaxed you feel good about yourself and your relationships, and you prob-ably have an optimistic attitude towards life and your future – all things that provide a positive framework in which to conceive.

The art of relaxation

Build some relaxation into your life
Undertaking any of the exercises suggested in the chart on page 108 will help you to relax, but being able to relax at will is useful not only through-

Muscle relaxation

When stress builds up over a period of time, you may find that your muscles become tense, stiff and painful. One way to relieve built-up muscle tension is to tense and relax each muscle in your body progressively. Combined with deep, controlled breathing, the more frequently you perform this relaxation technique the easier you will find it to enter into a state of deep relaxation. To practice muscle relaxation, follow the steps below:

1 Wearing warm, comfortable clothing, lie down on the floor or lie back in a comfortable chair. Breathe deeply and slowly for a few minutes until you have established a regular, relaxed breathing pattern. If you can, have someone pick up your arm or leg and drop it gently to check that you are properly relaxed.

2 Puff out your cheeks, then blow the air slowly out of your mouth. Puff out your abdomen with a deep breath then exhale slowly. Repeat this five times.

3 Trying not to use any other muscles in your body, bring your shoulders up to your ears and then relax them Repeat this five times.

4 Make tight fists and hold this for ten seconds, then relax them. Repeat this also five times.

5 Breathing evenly all the while, tense the muscles in your toes for a few seconds by curling up your foot. Then slowly relax them. Again, repeat this five times.

6 Using the same technique, tense and relax the rest of your body. Start with your ankles, calves and thighs, then abdomen, chest, hands, arms and your face.

out pregnancy and labour, but in all sorts of anxiety-inducing situations, from sitting in the dentist's chair to waiting for your child's first appearance in the school play! Relaxation helps you to get rid of muscle tension, slow down your heart rate and breathing, and gradually feel more at ease. It can also protect your body from the damaging effects of continuous stress. You may be surprised to discover that relaxation is an art that can be learned. Most relaxation exercises can be performed almost anywhere and at any time, and you will find them most beneficial if you learn to recognise signs of tension and then practice active relaxation regularly, not just when you have reached the end of your fuse.

There are many different relaxation techniques, the majority of which teach you how to relax individual muscle groups and control your breathing. The relaxation techniques that are taught for labour and birth (such as the Lamaze technique) can also be used during times of stress or you might also like to consider learning the Alexander Technique.

According to Frederick Matthias Alexander (1869–1955), the man who developed the Alexander Technique, the way we move is generally so inefficient and awkward that muscular tension builds up, causing all sorts of joint pains and stress disorders. By learning how to move correctly, you can release muscular tension, improve the way you breathe and reduce physical stress. It is almost impossible to do this yourself, however, so the Alexander Technique requires qualified teachers to help you reeducate your body through one-to-one tuition, often with the use of music.

Yoga also offers a great way to relax by combining stretching with controlled breathing and meditation. There are many styles or schools of yoga but the stretching postures all provide valuable physical release for tension, while the meditation stills the mind. You can meditate on positive thoughts, a helpful prayer or scripture.

T'ai chi, another relaxation system originating in the East, also combines slow, precise movements with a meditative state of mind. The smooth, snakelike movements are a useful form of muscle control and help both to exercise and relax various parts of the body. T'ai chi is a part of everyday life in many Chinese societies and this cultural acceptance of the need for relaxation has been particularly helpful in fast-moving, modern-

In many Asian societies, it is common to see t'ai chi being practiced by large groups of people in public, open spaces.

paced countries such as Taiwan where, despite the long working hours, people still find the time to practice t'ai chi. In any park, square or street corner in Taiwan, it is not uncommon to see individuals of all ages squatting or poised on one leg as they concentrate on moving slowly through t'ai chi routines while heavy traffic rushes by. For more information about the Alexander Technique, yoga or t'ai chi turn to Useful Addresses on page 187.

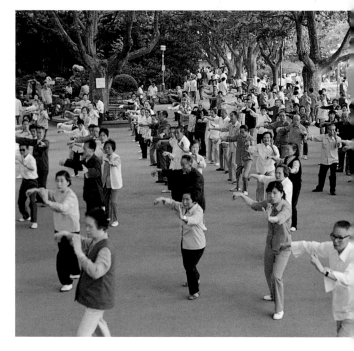

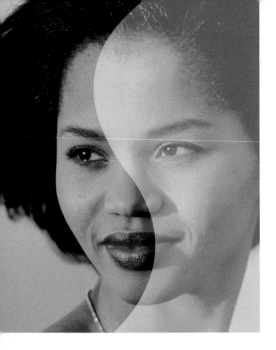

Quitting Bad Habits

We all know that smoking cigarettes, drinking too much alcohol and using drugs for social reasons are bad for our general health. But when it comes to fertility and conception, not only is your own health at risk, many of these habits will also affect your baby's health – at birth and throughout childhood. Deciding to become a parent is the time to take a long, hard look at your use of any of these social "props," and free yourself from their toxic effects.

The dangers of smoking

You may have first smoked a cigarette out of curiosity or because of peer pressure, but you probably had no idea how easily it could become a habit and how serious a hazard it is to your health. Not only does smoking have unattractive side effects – your hair and clothes smell of smoke, your fingers and teeth become stained, and your skin starts to wrinkle prematurely – it also reduces the length of your fertile years.

As well as the infamous and addictive nicotine and the carcinogenic compound tar, tobacco smoke contains thousands of deadly poisons, including arsenic, cyanide and carbon monoxide. These toxic substances damage your body in a number of ways: they constrict the small blood vessels in your body, restricting your blood flow and increasing your blood pressure; they act as mutagens, causing faulty cell division that can lead to cancer; they compromise the body's immune system, leaving you more prone to disease and infection; and they decrease the production of hormones, especially oestrogen, which may disrupt your fertility. The carcinogenic substances in tobacco smoke can cause lung cancer, as well as increase the risk of cancer of the cervix, mouth, throat, bladder, stomach and liver, to name but a few. Smokers are also more likely to die prematurely of heart disease, chronic bronchitis and emphysema.

On average, one in two regular smokers will eventually be killed by their habit and the majority of these won't live long enough to collect their old age pensions. The good news is that if you stop smoking before you develop any of these deadly diseases, your risk starts to drop right away. Research shows that after ten years of not smoking, your lifelong risk of developing most smoking-related diseases is the same as that of other non-smokers.

Smoking and female fertility

Traditionally, smoking was a male-dominated habit, but in the past few decades, many young girls started taking up the habit in an attempt to look "cool." About 30 per cent of young girls smoke and more girls under the age of 16 are likely to be regular smokers than boys of that same age.

Female smokers tend to have lower oestrogen levels than nonsmokers. This seems to be because the granulosa cells surrounding each ovum are inhibited by cigarette toxins. Low oestrogen levels may fail to stimulate the release of adequate amounts of LH, and this can prevent ovulation from occurring. Female smokers may also have poor quality cervical mucus.

Smoking may have a direct effect on the hypothalamus and pituitary gland. Along with lowered oestrogen levels, this can make female smokers prone to menstrual irregularities. Even if they do ovulate regularly, nicotine and other cigarette toxins can still reduce the chance of fertilisation by making ova impenetrable to sperm. These effects mean that nonsmokers are twice as likely as smokers to become pregnant within a year of trying. Smoking can also shorten a woman's reproductive life – heavy smokers tend to reach the menopause several years early. As fertility tends to decline sharply in the ten years leading up to the menopause, this could mean that the fertility of a 35-year-old smoker may be equivalent to that of a 40-year-old nonsmoker.

If you are a smoker you can increase your fertility and your chances of a successful conception from the moment you stop or significantly cut down the amount of cigarettes you smoke. (For tips to help you quit, turn to page 130.) Even if you are in the early stages of pregnancy, don't feel that it's too late to stop smoking. When it comes to improving your health, it's always better late than never!

If you cannot give up smoking, increase your intake of foods rich in vitamins A, C and E (see pages 92–95 for good sources). These help counteract the effects of smoking and encourage healthy sex cell production.

Smoking and male fertility

Around two in five men between the ages of 20 and 30 regularly smoke around 20 cigarettes a day, which can have devastating effects on male fertility. Men who smoke tend to have lower sperm counts than men who don't smoke. Also, the quality of sperm that male smokers produce is much poorer than those who don't, with more abnormal sperm of poorer motility. Because of Nature's inbuilt safety mechanism, low-quality sperm will rarely succeed in fertilising an ovum, but if they do, these sperm may carry hidden genetic defects, which can put the health of a pregnancy and baby at serious risk.

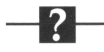

In 1983, the results of a large German research project into the risk factors in pregnancy was published. This study of nearly 8,000 births was one of the first to examine the effects of fathers' smoking habits during conception and pregnancy on their children's health. The results showed that fathers who smoked more than ten cigarettes a day during this time not only put their partners at increased risk of a miscarriage, but also put their newborn babies at increased risk of dying soon after birth as a result of prematurity, poor growth or life-threatening birth defects. Fortunately, the effects of smoking on sperm quality are reversible and the quality of a man's sperm should improve three months after he stops smoking.

Of all the births monitored in the German study, 2 in 100 babies born to smoking fathers suffered severe birth defects, compared to less than 1 in 100 born to nonsmoking fathers. These results indicated that the commonly quoted 2–3 in 100 risk of having a baby with a serious birth defect may be less if the parents do not smoke.

Passive smoking

Even if you don't smoke, you may still be exposed to other people's cigarette smoke at home, in the workplace or in public places. This is called passive smoking and can be as harmful as smoking small numbers of cigarettes yourself. In the UK it is estimated that over 500 nonsmokers die of lung cancer each year as a result of passive smoking.

If you are pregnant, your unborn baby has no choice but to suffer the effects of your breathing in smoke as well, and passive smoking when pregnant can lead to a reduction in your baby's birth weight. When you are planning to conceive you should protect your health and fertility by avoiding smoky places, and breathing in clean, fresh air instead. It is in all our interests to encourage nonsmoking offices, restaurants and public transport, and if your partner smokes you can help him to quit (see page 130). In the meantime, ask him and others who are smokers to smoke outdoors.

Long-term health risks for children of smokers

Sadly, the health risks for babies born to smokers do not end at birth, even if their parents stop smoking. Children whose mothers smoked in pregnancy are twice as likely as children of nonsmokers to suffer from respiratory problems such as bronchitis or asthma.

Recent research from the National Institute of Environmental Health in North Carolina, USA has suggested that there may be an increased risk of childhood cancers among the children of fathers who smoked before their conception. This was confirmed by a 1997 report published by the

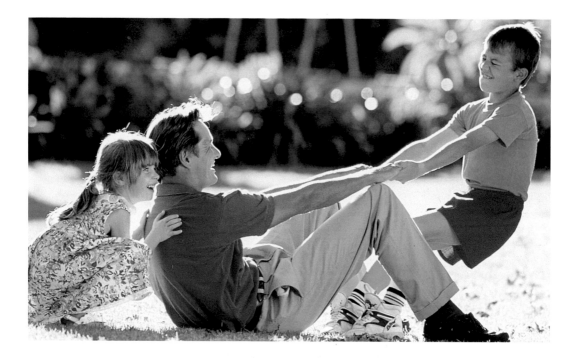

Oxford (UK) Study of Childhood Cancers, which also stated that children of fathers who smoke are at increased risk of developing various cancers in childhood. It should be pointed out, however, that childhood cancers such as leukemia are rare and although the risk is doubled for the children of heavy smokers, these cancers still only affect a small number of children.

By not smoking, especially in the preconception period, you and your partner will be ensuring the good health of your children.

Even if you manage to stop smoking in the preconception period and during pregnancy, don't think your job is over! Passive smoking is a serious threat to any child's health and it is estimated that one quarter of the risk of Sudden Infant Death Syndrome (SIDS: also known as Cot Death) in the first year of a baby's life is due to parental smoking. If you stay off cigarettes you will contribute to your family's good health in the long-term.

Time to stop

Now that you are planning a family you are probably in the best frame of mind to make the difficult but positive decision to curb your smoking. Who knows, this may be your chance finally to kick the habit – and for life! When you consider the health of your intended children you may find the extra motivation you need to go through the temporary deprivations of freeing yourself from this addiction. But remember, it's not just your baby's health that you will be protecting – you are worth it too, and breaking your dependency will improve your own health, now and in the future.

Smoking during pregnancy

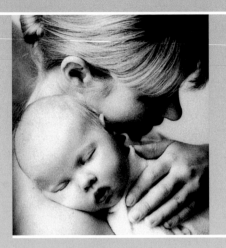

About one in three women of childbearing age in the UK is a smoker, yet less than one in ten give up during pregnancy. This is despite the fact that women who smoke during pregnancy have an increased risk of spontaneous abortion, bleeding in pregnancy, premature rupture of the membranes (which can lead to infection and premature birth), and of giving birth to a low birth weight baby.

Dangers for developing babies

A woman who smokes during her pregnancy can starve her unborn baby of oxygen and essential nutrients, and this can prevent her baby from growing properly. This is because the nicotine in cigarette smoke constricts the blood vessels in the placenta, and the carbon monoxide enters the baby's bloodstream, replacing some of the valuable oxygen molecules carried by haemoglobin in the red blood cells.

Some poisons from cigarette smoke, such as carbon monoxide, actually circulate in higher quantities in the baby's bloodstream than in the mother's. This is because a foetus cannot breathe smoke out again and has to wait for the placenta to clear it. These effects account for the fact that, on average, babies born to smoking mothers are at least half a pound underweight — a sign that they have been undernourished in the uterus — and may be more susceptible to infection at birth.

Dangers for pregnant women

Smoking during pregnancy can also be a serious health risk for mothers-to-be. To compensate for the reduced blood supply, the placenta tends to overgrow and may become detached from the uterus before the end of a woman's pregnancy. This is known as placental abruption and is a serious condition which can cause life-threatening bleeding for the mother-to-be and baby.

Placenta praevia (where the placenta implants too low in the uterus and can overlie the cervix) is also more common among women who smoke during their pregnancies. In this position the placenta can become detached in early labour and can cause heavy bleeding. In such instances, an emergency caesarean section is usually needed.

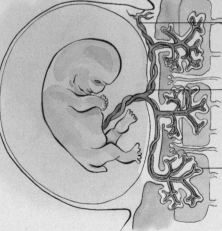

Umbilical veins (red) carry oxygenated blood back to foetus.

Umbilical arteries (blue) carry deoxygenated blood to placenta to receive oxygen.

Exchange between maternal and foetal blood.

A chance encounter holds the key

Hillary, a regular smoker, was 27 years old and worked as a bank clerk. She and her boyfriend Peter had been trying for a baby for the last 18 months but with no success.

"Until Peter and I decided to start a family, I hardly noticed how irregular my periods were. After 18 months of trying and still no pregnancy, I decided to keep a diary. I soon discovered that my periods only came every five or six weeks and were always very light. I was drinking alcohol only very occasionally, so I couldn't see what was causing it.

One day I ran into an old college friend who was working as a nurse. As we were chatting, she mentioned that my smoking could be affecting my periods. Although I wasn't allowed to smoke at work, I managed to get through 20 cigarettes a day during coffee breaks and in the evenings. I had never supposed that smoking could affect my ability to get pregnant, but I had promised myself I would quit once a baby was on its way.

After that chance meeting, I decided to tackle my habit sooner rather than later and made the effort to give up. Peter has never smoked and was a great support during that time.

After I quit smoking, I put on a bit more weight, my periods became more frequent, and three months later I finally conceived! I was so glad that I quit and I don't think I'll ever start again."

Some people find they can stop smoking overnight. If you are one of them, then congratulations! Keep it up. If you are smoking more than ten a day you are probably physically addicted as well as psychologically hooked, so when you quit expect to feel worse before you feel better. For example, your cough may worsen as the tiny cilia (hairs) in your lungs, which were paralysed by cigarette smoke, start to carry out all the rubbish accumulated in your lungs over the years. You may also find your sleep is disturbed and you feel irritable or tired. However, take these signs as encouragement that your body is re-adjusting from the poisonous effects of cigarette smoking. The worst physical withdrawal symptoms usually subside within two to three weeks. If you can cut your consumption by half before you stop completely, you may suffer fewer side effects. But don't kid yourself that you will eventually get down to one a day and then stop – you will still need to set a day to actually quit the habit altogether. For practical steps to quit smoking, see the box above.

Cutting down on alcohol

For thousands of years civilizations as different as the Greeks and Jews recommended that women should abstain from drinking alcohol around the time of conception. In the Bible Samson's mother was given the following

How to quit smoking

Before you can give up smoking, you need to convince yourself it's worth it, and the first step is finding out (and believing) the harm it causes. Once you see just how important it is to stop, use the following visualisation whenever you feel like a cigarette: picture your child growing in your uterus, healthy and free of all the toxic effects of cigarettes. Here is a plan to help you quit:

- Set a date to stop smoking altogether. Mark the date in your diary and tell someone else about it.
- Throw away all the smoking paraphernalia, such as lighters and ash trays, that remind you of smoking.
- Plan to buy something with the money you will save each week from not buying cigarettes.
- Work out which situations make you light up (a coffee after a meal), and make sure you have some sugar-free gum to put in your mouth instead of a cigarette.
- Get some support – your partner, a friend, a support group, so that you are not alone.
- Learn a relaxation technique (see page 121) and exercise more. This way, when you feel stressed you won't feel that smoking a cigarette is the only way out.

advice, "You are sterile and childless, but you are going to conceive and have a son. Now see to it that you drink no wine or other fermented drink." (Judges 13 vv 3,4.) And commenting on the gin-soaked poverty of England in the 18th century, the Royal College of Physicians of that day reported that children born to alcoholic parents were weak, feeble and underweight.

Couples today who are planning to start a family are still advised to moderate their drinking habits, but instead of this advice being based on folklore, there is now valid scientific research to back up these claims. Not only do we have a better understanding of the effects of alcohol on men and women who are planning to become parents, we also know the effects alcohol can have on babies during pregnancy.

How alcohol is metabolised
Alcohol is absorbed from the stomach into the bloodstream and passes into all parts of your body. Some alcohol is stored in fat cells and released later, which is one reason why women (who have a higher fat content than men) are often affected by alcohol for longer than men. In the liver, alcohol is broken down by an enzyme called alcohol dehydrogenase (men have more of this enzyme than women, another reason why they can consume greater amounts of alcohol and process it more quickly than women). Alcohol is then converted to acetaldehyde, which can eventually be used by the body to make energy. Acetaldehyde is poisonous to a developing baby.

Alcohol has an anaesthetic effect, slowing down messages from your brain and along your nerves. Although this can make you feel relaxed or unin-hibited, your reactions will immediately be slower and you may say or do things you wouldn't otherwise. The effects of alcohol start before any of the well-known signs of drunkenness, such as slurred speech. Your judge-ment while driving, for instance, is impaired however little you drink.

The toxic effects of alcohol can affect the ability of men and women to produce healthy sperm and ova. In the testes and ovaries alcohol interferes with the delicate process of cell division, just as the chromosomes are being sorted and separated, a time when accuracy is so important.

The effects of alcohol on male fertility

Although some men seem to be able to drink alcohol without any serious effects on their fertility, alcohol can have very damaging effects on sperm production: drinking alcohol depresses the hormone levels sent out from the pituitary and hypothalamus glands so that testosterone and sperm pro-duction levels fall. The toxins in alcohol also have a direct effect on the testes, disrupting the division of sperm cells.

Titled "Gin Lane," this 18th-century engraving by British artist William Hogarth reflects the time when doctors began to realise that "weak and sickly" babies were usually born to alcoholic mothers.

On average, men who drink four units of alcohol a day run the risk of having a lowered sperm count. Also, high numbers (sometimes more than 50 per cent) of the sperm that they do produce can be abnormal. Although this still leaves plenty of apparently normal sperm, these may not be fully motile. In time, alcoholic men eventually suffer from testicular atrophy and low testosterone levels, so sperm production may fail altogether.

Even if sperm production is not affect-ed, the short-term effects of alcohol can impair the sperms' ability to reach the ovum successfully – sperm are simply too drunk to find their way up the Fallopian tubes! A more practical problem for men who drink excessively is that they may find it difficult to perform sexually due to erectile problems. So, far from being a macho drink, alcohol can lead to impotence.

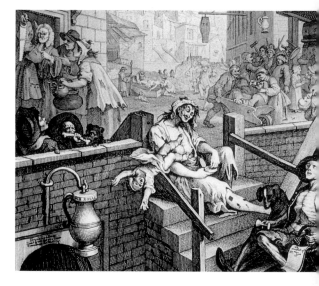

Any man hoping to father a child should, ideally, stop drinking alcohol on a regular basis for at least three months prior to conception to allow healthy sperm to develop. But stopping even for just a month before conception can improve your chances

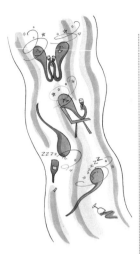

of successful fertilisation. Research conducted by Dr Marsha Morgan at the Royal Free Hospital in London, UK showed that men drinking two to four units of beer a day (that's only one or two pints!) can suffer from alcohol-related semen abnormalities. In her group of nearly 70 men experiencing fertility problems, 40 per cent began to show an improvement in their sperm quality just one month after they stopped drinking.

The effects of alcohol on female fertility

Alcohol depresses the hypothalamus gland and reduces the levels of stimulating hormones, which may interfere with ovulation. The main damage alcohol causes to female fertility, however, is its ability to disturb the delicate process of meiosis (see page 18).

Although heavy drinking can prevent ovulation, it's not common. For most women, drinking moderately will not prevent them from conceiving and even alcoholic women are not usually infertile as a result of alcohol. However, once conception has occurred drinking alcohol can cause a pregnancy to fail in several ways. The earliest problem can be that the fertilised ovum does not implant, possibly because the corpus luteum fails to produce enough progesterone and the luteal phase is cut short. Without enough progesterone (the hormone responsible for sustaining a pregnancy until the placenta forms) a pregnancy cannot be established.

A little later in pregnancy, drinking even only moderate amounts of alcohol can increase your chance of miscarriage. In 1980 Harlap and Shiono, two obstetricians working in Jerusalem, Israel, followed the drinking habits of over 32,000 women throughout their pregnancies. The results of their survey showed that women who drank as little as one to two units of alcohol a day (a unit is defined below) ran twice the risk of losing their pregnancy through miscarriage compared to women who didn't drink at all. Those who drank over three units a day were more than three times as likely to miscarry as those who did not drink at all. Other studies confirm

Drinking more than one unit of alcohol a day can increase a woman's risk of miscarriage. One unit of alcohol is equivalent to the following:

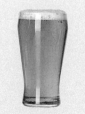

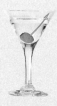

Half a pint of beer
(284 ml or 10 fl oz)

A glass of wine
(85 ml or 3 fl oz)

A measure of spirits
(25 ml or ¼ fl oz)

An aperitif
(50 ml or 2 fl oz)

LOOKING AHEAD Drinking during pregnancy

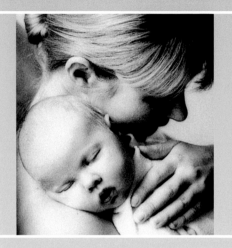

The effects of alcohol last longer in pregnancy. This is partly because its absorption from the gut wall becomes slower and also because some alcohol is stored in fat and released later, and fat stores increase in pregnancy.

After a drink, alcohol is distributed around the body and passes into tissues containing water. A pregnant woman carries an extra 6 litres (10½ pints) of water in tissue fluids, giving alcohol much more room to be distributed in, which can make her feel less effect from a drink. But even if you have a high tolerance of alcohol, don't make the mistake of thinking that your baby will have a similar tolerance.

Any alcohol that a mother drinks while she is pregnant will cross the placenta and pass on to her baby. Just like his mother, an unborn baby will only be able to get rid of alcohol by breaking it down with enzymes in

the liver. Unfortunately, a young foetus has no liver until it is about eight weeks old and, even then, it is very immature and incapable of converting alcohol as efficiently as a fully developed liver. As a result, the foetus takes about twice as long as his mother to be free of the effects of any alcohol she drinks.

During pregnancy, it's sensible to avoid spirits and to limit your alcohol intake to a maximum of only one unit a day (see page 132). Try to get into the habit of drinking soft drinks instead.

the link between moderate alcohol intake and miscarriage, particularly in the second trimester of pregnancy, when most women feel they are past the risk of miscarriage.

The links between drinking alcohol and miscarriage may also be partly due to poor nutrition. Alcoholic drinks tend to provide calories in the form of sugar and alcohol, but without the vitamins needed to metabolise them. Also, because alcoholic drinks are filled with calories and therefore satisfy your appetite, women who drink a lot tend to eat less of the nutrient-rich food that they need to stay healthy.

So can you safely drink at all around the time of conception?

The easy answer to this question is no! Because alcohol has no known benefits for fertility, the only absolutely safe limit for future parents is none.

FOETAL ALCOHOL SYNDROME

Mothers who drink heavily during pregnancy are prone to giving birth to babies with a group of serious health problems that are known together as foetal alcohol syndrome (FAS).

Babies born with this syndrome tend to be small with poorly developed heads, small eyes and jaws, and may suffer from birth defects including heart problems, genital malformations and limb defects. They may also be irritable, have feeding and breathing difficulties, and trouble sleeping. Sadly, these effects are not temporary and continue into adult life. Because of a deficiency in growth hormones these children may also grow up to be short in stature and have learning difficulties as a result of low IQ. Although not all babies of mothers who drink habitually will develop all the signs and problems of FAS, it is thought that most infants born to mothers drinking more than five units a day will be affected in some way, and one in three of these will have the full FAS. The syndrome probably affects one in ten babies born to women regularly drinking three units a day. The syndrome rarely develops in babies whose mothers drink less than ten units a week during pregnancy.

Yet having said this, it's very unlikely that one alcoholic drink a day will affect your fertility or increase your risk of miscarriage.

The important thing to avoid is drinking regularly or heavily (or binge drinking) at any one time. Although the recommended safe intake of alcohol for women is seven units a week, this does not mean that drinking seven units in one evening is safe. Men should avoid drinking more than two units a day in the months leading up to and around the time of conception, and they should keep their intake down to 10 to 14 units a week. Eating a healthy diet (see chapter 6: Food for Fertility) may help to protect you from the effects of alcohol and never drink on an empty stomach as this speeds up absorption.

The hazards of drugs

Whether legal or illegal, all drugs are by definition foreign chemicals to the body that could be potentially hazardous for fertility or the development of an unborn baby. Even caffeine in excess may affect your fertility (see page 96). Obviously, some drugs are safer than others and all licensed drugs are extensively tested before being approved for prescription. However, the memory of the teratogenic effects of thalidomide should remind us that all women need to be very cautious and only take necessary medication during pregnancy and around the time of conception under the supervision of a doctor. For a list of some of the more commonly prescribed medications and their known effects on fertility and pregnancy see pages 170–71.

Drugs affect people according to how well their liver can produce enzymes to break them down and how much body fat they have. A person's nutritional state is also important and the poorly nourished tend to excrete drugs very slowly. The effects of misused illegal drugs on the foetus are difficult to study because often men and women who are dependent on drugs may also have poor diets, smoke cigarettes and drink alcohol. Similarly, long-term effects on children whose mothers consumed illegal drugs during pregnancy can also be hard to monitor as they are frequently born into homes with social problems that tend to have an adverse effect on their development. However, most illegal drugs can seriously damage your fertility or your unborn baby.

DRUGS AND YOUR FERTILITY

There is no evidence to suggest that previous drug abuse among healthy adults will affect the development of their unborn babies. However, if you currently use drugs and plan to conceive, try to seek help now to stop before pregnancy.

Drug	Effect
Cannabis	Similar to smoking; damaged sperm production, increased risk of placental abruption during pregnancy, premature and low birth-weight babies.
Opiates	Damaged sperm production, chance of conceiving non-identical twins increases threefold, poor foetal growth, premature birth, and risk of sudden death after birth.
Cocaine	Similar to moderate alcohol intake; birth defects, low birth-weight and undernourished at birth. Exposure in utero may cause psychiatric problems in childhood.
Amphetamines	Menstrual irregularities and poor fertility.
Tranquillizers	Newborn breathing difficulties, depressed nervous system.

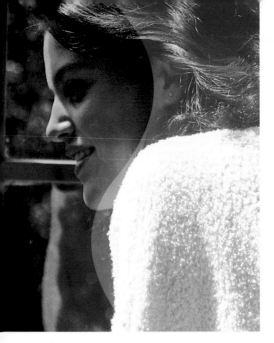

Avoiding Environmental Hazards

In addition to personal health issues such as diet, fitness, and medication, your surrounding environment also can have an effect on your fertility. Exposure to radiation and chemicals are the main environmental hazards for future parents at home and in the workplace. But far from being out of your control, it is possible to eliminate or reduce your exposure to these hazards once you become aware of them.

The risks from radiation

Radiation is a general term that is used to describe the energy waves of the electromagnetic spectrum. These waves are distinguished by their lengths and frequencies (the shorter the wavelength, the higher the frequency). At one end of the spectrum are the high-energy, potentially damaging ionising rays, such as cosmic rays, x-rays and UV rays. At the other end of the spectrum are the safer, low-energy, low-frequency non-ionising waves, such as radio waves and microwaves. In the middle of the spectrum is optical radiation, which includes visible light (see the diagram on right).

We are all exposed to some radiation every day of our lives. Natural sources of radiation include cosmic rays from the sky, radon gas from the ground and radioactive potassium in our food. Other sources of non-ionising electromagnetic radiation include power lines, microwave ovens, mobile telephones, computers and even the television.

The effects of radiation on fertility

Not all radiation is known to be harmful and it is mainly exposure to the emissions of ionising radiation (radioactivity) and ultraviolet (UV) light that is the major health risk. Prolonged exposure to UV light damages skin cells, which can cause skin cancer, but the light does not penetrate far enough into the body to affect the reproductive system. Ionising radiation, on the other hand, can damage dividing cells inside the body, which puts the sperm, ova and blood cells at high risk.

In high doses ionising radiation will kill any cell outright, but lower doses are still dangerous. Exposure to radiation can damage the genetic material in the nucleus of a cell and this can lead to mistakes when that cell divides. Many animal experiments have shown that exposure of a freshly released or newly fertilised ovum to x-rays can cause chromosome damage and lead to miscarriage. If the affected cells are already part of a tiny, developing foetus, organs may not develop properly and this can lead to birth defects. In adults and children radiation may cause susceptibility to infection or lead to cancers, such as leukemia, developing unchecked by the body's immune system.

Sources of ionising radiation

Radiation is measured in millisieverts and in the UK, each person is exposed to an average ionising radiation dose of two and a half millisieverts annually. In the US each person is exposed to an average ionising radiation dose of one millisievert annually. Exposure to radioactivity can be potentially danger-ous, but the acceptable annual dose limit set by the UK government for workers in radio-active industries is 50 mil-lisieverts, although very few get anywhere near this level of exposure.

In the UK and US, radon gas from the ground is the single biggest source of natural radiation and makes up half the average yearly exposure a person has to ionising radiation. It can accumulate in buildings through cracks in the foundation, basement and floors. A person's exposure to radon has been linked to a small increase in the risk of developing lung cancer and leukemia, but evidence of its specific effects at the time of conception is scarce.

If you think you might live in a high-risk area (certain areas are known to be high-risk) the Environmental Protection Agency (EPA) will be able to advise you on what kind of pro-tective building measures you can take, for example, improving the ventilation in your home to draw out radon from beneath its foundations. You may want to consider having your house treated in this way, or even moving before you decide to try and start a family. This may help to prevent your children from being exposed to radon as they grow up.

Gamma rays from the ground and buildings contribute another unavoidable 14 per cent of the average person's yearly radiation exposure. Cosmic rays from space can contribute around ten per cent, but if you live at high altitude or travel a

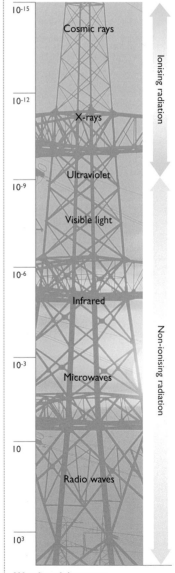

There are many types of waves on the electromagnetic spectrum. High-frequency, ionising waves, such as x-rays, pose a greater risk to fertility than low-frequency, non-ionising waves, such as radio waves.

10^{-15}

Cosmic rays

Ionising radiation

10^{-12}

X-rays

Ultraviolet

10^{-9}

Visible light

10^{-6}

Infrared

Non-ionising radiation

10^{-3}

Microwaves

10

Radio waves

10^{3}

Wavelength in metres

PARENTAL EXPOSURE TO RADIATION AND CHILDHOOD LEUKEMIA – IS THERE A LINK?

The life-threatening effects of radiation have been well documented since radioactivity was first studied at the end of the 19th century, but it has since been harder to prove any link between exposure of parents to low levels of ionising radiation around the time of conception, and problems among their children, for example birth defects and cancers.

In 1994, doctors from the University of Minnesota published a study of 300 children with leukemia. It showed a link between the fathers' exposure to abdominal x-rays around the time of their children's conception, and the risk of their children developing the cancer. But there was no clear link between the mothers' exposure to x-rays and leukemia in their children.

In 1990 Dr Gardner and his colleagues reporting to the Health and Safety Executive in the UK published data on an unexpected group of children suffering from leukemia whose fathers were exposed to ionising radiation at the Sellafield nuclear plant in the north-west of England before the children were conceived. Since then, larger studies throughout the UK have shown a similar link, but they have also shown, rather unexpectedly, that fathers with high-level exposure were less likely than men with low-level exposure to have an affected child. The increased risk of miscarriage following high-level exposure may account for this. For example, far fewer babies were born between seven and nine months after the Hiroshima bombing than expected, probably because of fatal damage sustained at the time of the explosion around conception.

Overall, mothers who worked in the nuclear power industry did have children with a small increased risk of childhood cancers, but most of the risk appeared to be due to their exposure during pregnancy, not before the time of conception. Even the children of parents exposed to ionising radiation preconceptionally in the Japanese atomic bombings did not show an inherited leukemia risk. Also, men who have had radiation treatment for testicular cancer and who have gone on to have children do not seem to pass on a risk of childhood cancer (most, however, would have been rendered infertile by the treatment, so these represent an unusual group of fathers).

At present, it seems as if something apart from exposure to ionising radiation may explain the findings in these studies.

lot by plane, this can be much higher. On average, aircrew are exposed to an extra two millisieverts a year, which puts them in a similar category of extra exposure to nuclear industry workers. Ten hours in the air is equivalent to having a chest x-ray.

About 12 per cent of ionising radiation comes from food and water and cannot be easily avoided, except by avoiding foods from known high-risk areas, for example, where seafood may be contaminated by waste water from the nuclear power industry. Non-natural sources of ionising radiation include diagnostic medical x-rays, which make up about 12 per cent of the average person's exposure to radiation. An abdominal x-ray gives about one and a half millisieverts of radiation and a chest x-ray only 0.05 millisieverts.

Today, some x-rays can be avoided by using magnetic resonance imaging (MRI), which gives almost negligible doses of ionising radiation. Other scanning techniques, such as ultrasound, can also be used more safely than x-rays. This is why ultrasound scans and not x-rays are used in pregnancy. In fact, x-rays are used very rarely during pregnancy. A course of radio-therapy used in cancer treatment would far exceed the total exposure from all other sources and such treatment would never be considered safe enough to use during pregnancy or around the time of conception.

Surprisingly, nuclear power accounts for only 0.1 per cent of a person's average total exposure to ionising radiation. Although this can rise to 0.3 millisieverts for people living near a processing plant, it is still far less than radiation from radon, and even the average nuclear industry worker receives only an extra two millisieverts a year. It is only when there is a serious accident, such as the Chernobyl disaster in 1986, that nuclear power plants present a grave risk. The remaining two per cent of our ionising radiation exposure is made up of fallout from luminous materials, exposure to television and radio-activity in the atmosphere from nuclear bomb testing and nuclear accidents.

Restricting your exposure to harmful radiation Your exposure to potentially harmful radiation may be increased if you travel a lot in aeroplanes, undergo medical x-rays, or work in the production or handling of radioactive chemicals. Unless you work in a high-risk occupation (see page 149), the best way you can reduce unnecessary exposure to ionising radiation is to avoid having medical x-rays near the time of conception and perhaps to limit non-essential air travel.

Stress and overwork are far more likely to affect reproductive health than radiation from visual display units (VDUs), which are considered safe to use during the pre-conception period.

Are you at risk from your domestic appliances?

So far the discussion has been about ionising radiation, but what about non-ionising radiation? In contrast to ionising radiation, the electromagnetic waves from domestic appliances, such as microwaves, cell phones and visual display units (VDUs), tend to be lower in energy and are not thought to cause damage to the genetic information carried in cells. Colour televisions do emit tiny amounts of radioactivity, as well as non-ionising radiation, but this is not enough to be dangerous.

In the late 1980s, there were a few alarming reports of high rates of miscarriage among women working with VDUs in America. However, further scientific investigation of much larger groups in America and Europe, did not show a risk. The apparent link between VDU work and miscarriage was thought to be due to stress at work and a recall bias among the women – women who have problems in pregnancy tend to report more possible risk factors in questionnaires than those women who experience healthy pregnancies and give birth to healthy babies.

Other sources of non-ionising radiation, such as overhead powerlines, have been investigated because of concerns that they might cause cancer, yet no link has been proved. There is certainly no evidence that living near such sources affects a man or woman's fertility, or the outcome of a pregnancy. In 1988, a study of female welders exposed to non-ionising radiation did not show any increased risk of their babies having birth defects or being stillborn.

Heat exposure

Sperm are very sensitive to heat, so heat exposure is a particular hazard for male fertility. The testes need to be cooler than the rest of the body to produce healthy sperm, which is why they hang outside the body in the scrotum. Even small increases in the temperature of the scrotum can reduce a man's sperm count, and prolonged heat exposure can result in infertility due to poor sperm count. Women are not vulnerable to heat in the same way, because the ovaries lie deep in their pelvis where the body temperature is kept constant during normal health. There is evidence to suggest that heat exposure during early pregnancy from saunas or a prolonged fever may increase the risk of birth defects, such as spina bifida, but this risk is probably very small.

There are a number of occupations that involve exposure to heat and these include welding, firefighting, working in bakeries, industrial laundries or engine rooms on board ship. If your partner works in one of these jobs he should take cool breaks in the open air, wear loose, cool clothing, and have a cool shower after work. Long hours behind a desk and jobs involving many hours of driving have also been linked with lower sperm counts as a result of overheating (see also Did You Know? on page 105), although a lack of exercise may also contribute to the problem.

Chemical hazards

The production of chemicals this century has mushroomed – pesticides, herbicides and synthetic hormones are manufactured for use in agriculture; plastics and polymers have been manufactured to replace many natural materials used in textiles, furniture and packaging; and the phar-

If you can't stand the heat...

William and Alison were both in their early 20s when they decided to try for a baby. Alison had always had regular periods and she and William were both in excellent health. So, when Alison had still not conceived after 18 months, they were a bit surprised and confused, and decided to go to their GP for advice.

"When we were called into our GP's surgery to discuss the results of our tests, our doctor explained to us that William's semen analysis showed he had a very low sperm count, with poor motility and a high proportion of abnormal sperm.

Until that time we had never considered William's job in the bakery to be a problem. But as our doctor pointed out, he was exposed to very high tempera-

tures all day and rarely took a break outside. The fact that he went to work in tight jeans, then put his bakery overalls on top of them, added to the problem.

William decided to reduce his exposure to the heat at work by only wearing loose underclothes beneath his overalls. He made sure he took regular breaks outside the bakery and also had a cold shower when he got home from work.

Eight weeks later, we were very excited to see the results of some follow-up tests – they showed that William's sperm count had risen threefold and his sperm were twice as motile. Four months later, we were thrilled when a pregnancy test confirmed that I had conceived. We are now happily looking forward to the arrival of our baby."

maceutical industry has produced thousands of new chemicals for use in medicines. If you work with toxic chemicals you are probably aware of the risks these have to your general health. However, these chemicals are also widely used in the home in cleaning, gardening or "do-it-yourself" home maintenance products and you should be aware of their potential hazards.

Toxic chemicals can affect a woman's fertility by causing menstrual irregularities, and exposure to these chemicals during pregnancy can cause miscarriage or birth defects. This was confirmed by a nationwide study conducted in Finland by Dr Hemminki and a team of researchers, published in 1980. Out of 11,000 miscarriages suffered by women in Finland, he found that there was a slightly increased risk for women who worked in agriculture and chemical industries compared to similar women working in clerical jobs. Exposure to toxic chemicals also can affect a man's fertility, leading to loss of libido as well as poor sperm production and motility.

Pesticides

As well as being used in large-scale agricultural and horticultural industries, pesticides are also used in parks, in gardens, in homes for treating woodworm, and in medicines to treat lice and fleas. Unfortunately, they not only kill insects and fungi, but they may also damage human fertility.

DID YOU KNOW?

Sperm are so sensitive to heat that several types of contraceptive truss have been developed. These hold the testes tightly against the body so they cannot cool sufficiently for sperm manufacture. After using these for ten weeks or so, sperm counts dwindle to almost negligible amounts. These effective but uncomfortable devices don't look set to take the contraceptive market by storm, but they are now available in France, and well illustrate the devastating effect that heat can have on male fertility.

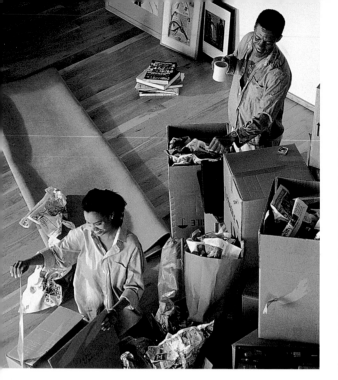

Pesticides that contain organochlorines (OCs – organic chlorine-containing chemicals) may act like oestrogen-like compounds (oestrogen, the female sex hormone, has the tendency to feminize male embryos and also to cause impotence and poor sperm production). Dieldrin, for example, is a herbicide found in weed killers and is known to cause sperm damage. Other pesticides known to damage male fertility include DDT. This was once used widely as an insecticide until the toxic effects were realised, and it is still used in some parts of the world to control the malarial mosquito. Kepone and lindane (see below) are two other dangerous pesticides.

If you are moving house, check it has been treated for woodworm and damp beforehand to avoid exposure to harmful chemicals. If this isn't possible, keep rooms well-ventilated and avoid conception until the risks subside.

Lindane is widely used as a wood preserver, for the treatment of woodworm, and is present in preparations that treat head lice and scabies. Repeated exposure to large doses can cause epileptic fits and aplastic anaemia (where red blood cells are not produced in sufficient quantities). Although most people are not affected in lower doses, pregnant women are nevertheless advised by the manufacturers of head lice and scabies preparations to avoid using them.

Many women catch head lice from their children, so if you are hoping to conceive, or are pregnant already, try an alternative to preparations containing lindane, for example, Pyrethrin. Regular use of shampoo and conditioner followed by combing with a nit comb has been shown to be just as effective in preventing head lice. If a medical treatment has been recommended, the compound permethrin is a safer alternative. Certain combinations of essential oils may also be effective in treating head lice, but ensure you consult a qualified aromatherapist who knows you are planning to conceive or may be pregnant.

DDT, lindane and dieldrin are very toxic pesticides and their use has been reduced in the UK since 1974, when a voluntary ban came into force. In the US, there is some restriction on the use of lindane in vapourized form and many countries, including Japan and Sweden, have banned its use altogether. Unfortunately, many pesticides are manufactured and used without any research being conducted into their possible reproductive hazards, and this is why there is very little information about the effects of many pesticides on female fertility.

Not all pesticides are as toxic as others and the people most at risk from exposure are those who work daily in pesticide-related industries. Because many foods contain pesticide residues, we are all exposed to small amounts in our food and water, although the impact on our health of such a small amount of exposure to pesticides is still unclear. However, when the London Food Commission carried out a survey in 1988 of all the pesticides currently permitted in the UK, it found that at least 35 had some unwanted effect on fertility and pregnancy, including impotence in men, miscarriage and birth defects. One way to reduce your exposure is to eat organically grown foods. Yet even these can contain some pesticides that have been carried by the wind or water from treated to untreated areas.

Heavy metals

Lead, mercury and cadmium are all toxic, heavy metals that are not naturally occurring in the body. Exposure to these metals can have a detrimental effect on male and female fertility.

Lead This was one of the first industrial chemicals to be recognised as a hazard to female fertility. In the UK, legislation was introduced in 1907 which prevented all women of childbearing age from working with lead in the paint industry. In the US, a worker's exposure to lead is regulated in many large-scale industries, but is still a problem in other industries such as battery manufacturing.

While most modern paints are now lead-free, lead-based paints may still be on old furniture. So, when stripping old paint, make sure you wear protective gloves and a mask.

Exposure to lead can cause sterility in both men and women, and can lead to miscarriage and stillbirth if the exposure occurs during pregnancy. Men and women can be exposed to lead fumes when using solder, especially in the electronics industry. Despite an increase in the number of vehicles running on lead-free petrol, petrol and exhaust fumes are still major sources of lead in the environment. Many countries have banned lead from being used in indoor paints, but other paints (particularly cheaper imported ones) may contain lead. If you are planning to strip down old paint that might contain lead, wear gloves and a mask, and consider delaying conception until three months after the job is finished.

Mercury Although mercury is a toxic metal, not many of us are exposed to high levels of it on a day-to-day basis. Amalgams (commonly used in dental fillings) contain high levels of mercury, so dental nurses and dentists can be at risk. If you need to have a tooth filled around the time you plan to conceive or when you are in the early weeks of pregnancy, you can ask your dentist to use a non-mercury compound, although this will be more expensive. You might also like to avoid having old mercury fillings removed around this time.

In men, exposure to organic mercury can decrease healthy sperm production; in women, it may affect their fertility through its toxic effects on the ovum. But it is during pregnancy that mercury poses the greatest risk: it can cause birth defects, and brain damage in an unborn baby seems to be a particular risk. Some weedkillers and cropdusts contain organic mercury compounds and exposure to these during pregnancy may also cause birth defects.

Cadmium This may cause poor sperm production in men and may cause infertility in women by interfering with the implantation of the fertilised egg into the lining of the uterus. Cigarettes are the main source of

Uncovering hidden risks at work

Maureen was 30 years old and working as a dental nurse when she found out she was expecting her first baby. Because she felt very healthy, she carried on working until her 35th week of pregnancy. However, three weeks later her son was stillborn and had signs of poor growth and brain damage.

"I was concerned during my pregnancy that the x-ray machine in the surgery was a possible risk to my baby, but I had always followed safety precautions really carefully. Nevertheless, the medical staff who delivered my baby suggested I got a risk assessment done at work before my next pregnancy. So I asked Graham, the dentist I worked for, to assess all the possible risks in the surgery because, despite my grief, I wanted to try for another baby as soon as it was safe.

The written risk assessment showed some surprising results. The x-ray machine was not considered a risk because both Graham and I left the room and operated it remotely, but the mercury levels in the surgery were considered hazardous. Because I was solely responsible for mixing dental amalgams, I had been exposed to high levels of mercury during my pregnancy. In the last two years we had also started using ethylene oxide instead of the traditional steam method to sterilise our equipment. The latest research showed that ethylene oxide gas can cause birth defects in animals and miscarriage and prematurity in human pregnancy, so this may have contributed to my stillbirth.

When I got pregnant again, Graham agreed to go back to using the old steriliser and also made up his own dental amalgams. (He was 53 and had already completed his family!) Again, I felt really healthy throughout my pregnancy, but took the precautionary measure of stopping work at 28 weeks of pregnancy to rest. Ten weeks later I gave birth to a healthy daughter."

cadmium, so when you are hoping to conceive you should try to avoid all exposure to cigarette smoke (see also Chapter 8). Cadmium is also used in electronic solder and some pesticides.

Other toxic metals Selenium is essential for fertility (see page 91) but very high doses of it can be toxic and could potentially damage a developing foetus. While you are unlikely to overdose on selenium from your diet, some hair treatments contain this metal.

Aluminum is not a highly toxic metal but there has been some slightly inconclusive evidence from animal experiments to suggest that it could cause birth defects. The main sources of aluminum are from cookware, anticaking agents in dried milk, and antacids used to treat indigestion. There is probably no cause for alarm about aluminium.

Solvents

Organic solvents are used in a wide variety of industries and many are known to have harmful effects on both the male and female reproductive systems. For instance, toluene, which is used in the shoe-making industry, has been shown to cause menstrual irregularities in 50 per cent of women and also can cause miscarriage. Tetrachloroethylene, which is found in dry-cleaning fluid, and benzene, which is used in the dye industry, shoe-making industry, and found in lead-free petrol, may both cause menstrual problems and damage to the unborn baby. Methylene chloride, which is found in paint stripper, has been shown to damage sperm production as well as cause menstrual problems and miscarriage.

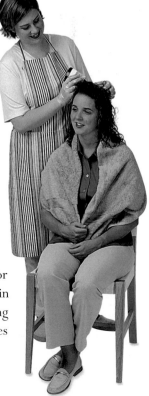

Many hair dyes contain selenium, a metal which can be toxic in high doses. So, when applying hair dyes, wear gloves.

Dioxins

These chemicals are produced as a by-product of chlorine bleaching, a technique used in the production of toilet paper, tea bags, sanitary towels and nappies. Some dioxins are particularly toxic and can be absorbed through our skin when we use these products, or taken in foods (for instance in milk from dioxin-contaminated milk cartons). As they tend to accumulate in fatty tissue, exposure to dioxins could, in theory, be particularly damaging when you are pregnant or breast-feeding because this is when fat stores may be used by the body for energy. At low levels of exposure, there is no evidence of damage in pregnancy abut research is lacking. Safety measures include choosing non chlorine-bleached paper products and buying milk in glass bottles instead of paper containers.

LOOKING AHEAD   The nesting instinct

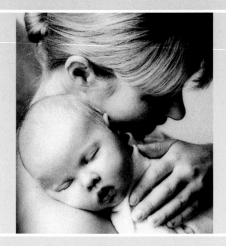

Once your pregnancy is well established you will probably want to plan your baby's nursery. However, you should be aware of the following guidelines for choosing the best furnishings and decorating safely during this time.

Not only will your baby sleep in the nursery, but you will also spend time feeding, changing and playing with her there. You'll therefore want to make sure that everything – from floor to ceiling – is safe for you and your baby.

If you are having any woodwork for the nursery treated, make sure you stay away from the area until the fumes and dust have subsided. If you plan to renovate old furniture, such as a wooden cot or a rocking chair, strip off the paint because it could contain lead and repaint with non-toxic, child-safe paint or varnish. If you are wallpapering the nursery, check that the paste you use is safe. The solvent in prepasted wallpaper is usually not toxic but as a precautionary measure, always

keep the room well-ventilated while you use any paint or paste with a nonwater-based solvent.

Research has suggested a link between a baby's bedding and sudden infant death syndrome (SIDS), so choose bedding carefully. Layers of natural fibre bedding, such as wool or cotton blankets are safer than synthetic quilts, which can cause a baby to overheat. Mattresses should be made to a high safety specification and have a safety approval marked. The latest research has not linked fire retardants on PVC mattresses with SIDS as once feared. If you are concerned about your baby developing allergies, opt for a polished floor with brightly coloured rugs (see also page 67).

Other hazardous chemicals

Many other chemicals with known reproductive hazards are used in a variety of manufacturing industries and your exposure to these should be avoided if you are planning to conceive or while you are pregnant. For instance, chloroprene is used in the manufacture of synthetic rubber and has been associated with infertility in men and women. Vinyl chloride and carbon disulfide are used in the manufacture of plastic and viscose, and can reduce libido and sperm production in men.

Women who work in operating theatres and are exposed to anaesthetic gases over prolonged periods may be at risk of losing a baby through miscarriage. Recent improvements in ducting waste gases out of the

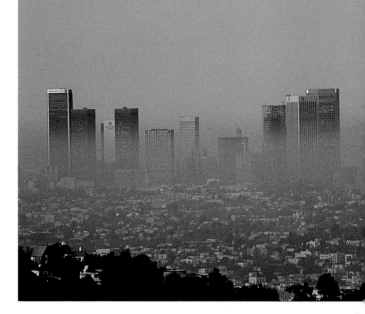

theatre have lowered the risk, but if in doubt, consider asking for a risk assessment of your own workplace. If you need an anaesthetic during pregnancy, the risks to your baby are probably very low, but obviously you should only have essential surgery during this time and put off any elective surgical treatment, such as for haemorrhoids, until after your baby is born.

Although polychlorinated biphenols (PCBs) are known to be toxic (and are now banned in the US), they are still used worldwide in a variety of industries, such as the manufacture of many exported transformers, inks, hydraulic fluids and degreasing agents in nuclear submarines.

Los Angeles is one modern city that is notorious for its smog. This is due to its unique climate and the high pollution caused by the city's traffic congestion.

PCBs can build up in fatty tissue because the body finds it very hard to get rid of them. They have had a high profile recently as they are thought to be causing feminising effects on many species of animals in areas where PCB pollution is high. For example, alligators in Lake Apopka, Florida have been known to undergo sex changes and polar bears in the Arctic have been sighted with hermaphrodite features. PCBs are persistent pollutants that remain in the environment for a long time and environmental lobbyists are now pressing for a worldwide ban on their use.

Pollution in the air

Although there is no evidence of air pollution being a risk for pregnancy, many of the toxic chemicals mentioned in this chapter can be found polluting our air, especially in urban areas or around industrial sites. Traffic fumes add lead, benzene, carbon monoxide and nitrous oxide to the air and many fuels release smoke containing sulphur dioxide when they are burned.

Air pollution varies considerably from day to day, hour to hour, and street to street. Where possible, avoid the streets during rush hour when the number of cars on the road increases pollution. If you are stuck in heavy traffic, try not to use your car heater, which draws air into the car from outside, and if you walk, choose routes that aren't crowded with queuing traffic. If your house is near a busy road, only open windows that are facing away from the traffic and use net curtains, which will help to filter the pollution.

How safe is your water?

Although drinking water in the UK is among the cleanest and safest in the world, toxic chemicals, such as lead from old pipes and nitrates from fertilisers in the soil, can contaminate the water supply. Water is regularly tested for around 60 chemicals, including lead, pesticide residues, bacteria and many other harmless minerals. If you are concerned about the quality of your water supply, you can request an analysis of your own tap water by your local water board. They should be able to tell you how the quality of your water compares to standard health guidelines. If you are worried about high levels of any chemical in your water, consider using a water filter or drinking mineral water, or replacing lead pipes.

Ensuring your health and safety at work

There are many hazards in the workplace that can be a health risk for pregnant women and their unborn babies. Although there is very little specific legislation protecting men and women from work hazards that might affect their fertility (except lead exposure), every employer, however small his workforce, has a responsibility to ensure your safety at work.

In practise this means that you have the right to have the type of work you do and your workplace assessed for any hazards, which must be explained to you. Your employer must provide you with any necessary safety equipment although it is your responsibility to use it. You should also be provided with reasonable rest periods to safeguard your health.

While some occupations are widely known to be potential causes of fertility problems (for instance, working with some toxic chemicals), others are less evident, but can nonetheless present some risk to your fertility. Noise, vibration and stress at work may all contribute to fertility problems. For example, there is some evidence that prolonged exposure to vibration can lead to menstrual irregularities and possibly female fertility problems. A woman exposed to whole body vibration, through working with heavy vibrating machinery in a factory, for example, may be at risk of mis-carriage or stillbirth.

You have the right to ask your employer for a written risk assessment of any possible hazards to your health, so if you are planning to conceive,this will include the effects that your work might have on your risk of miscarriage or birth defects in your baby. Risks may include obvious toxic hazards such as chemicals and radiation, but also heat exposure, standing for long hours, vibration and noise exposure. Once the risks of your job are known, your employer should take steps to provide you with the safety equipment you need to protect yourself and allow you to take proper rest breaks. It is then up to you to use the safety gear and carefully follow safety codes. For instance, if you work with chemicals you should wear gloves and protective clothing. If x-ray machines are used at work you should always wear your safety apron and stand behind the protective screens. Never get complacent and relax your safety measures – you may be putting the health of your future children at risk!

Once you are pregnant you will have added protection as you then have the right to ask for your working conditions to be altered in order to avoid potential health risks to you and your baby. This will be based on your risk assessment, so make sure you ask for this to be done in good time so you can prepare for your pregnancy. These work alterations could involve simple measures such as extra breaks if your work involves standing for long hours at a time, not lifting heavy objects or a complete change of environment if you work with or near dangerous chemicals. As your back is particularly vulnerable to strain in pregnancy you may be relieved of jobs involving lifting or operating heavy machinery.

ENVIRONMENTAL HAZARDS AND HIGH-RISK OCCUPATIONS

Depending on the everyday tasks your job involves, your risk of exposure to potentially dangerous environmental factors may be high or low. If you are in a high-risk occupation, make sure your employer gives you a written risk assessment so you can protect yourself during conception and pregnancy.

HAZARD	THOSE AT RISK
Ionizing radiation	Nuclear fuel workers, x-ray staff, miners, aircrew, workers confined to certain geographical areas.
Chemicals	Those in manufacturing, agricultural and horticultural jobs; dry-cleaning staff; laboratory technicians using chemical solvents; hairdressers (especially using dyes), anesthetists; dental staff. "Do-it-yourself" gardening, car maintenance and home renovation can also be hazardous.
Infection	Teachers, agricultural workers (particularly those who work with pregnant animals), nurses, doctors, and vets.
Physical stress	Anyone who performs physical work which could lead to injury or fatigue; e.g. nurses who do a lot of lifting, manual workers.
Noise and vibration	Operators of heavy vibrating machinery e.g. in car factories.
Heat exposure	Bakers, laundry workers, those in heavy manufacturing sector, anyone working in an engine room on board ship.
Travelling	Sales representatives.

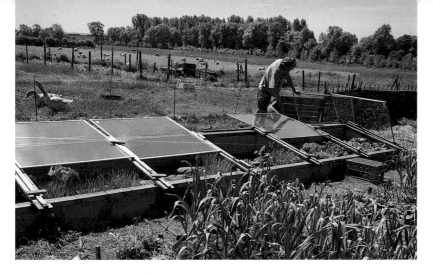

Organic farming methods have become increasingly popular because the resulting produce is free from artificial pesticides and other chemicals.

If your job is recognised as very hazardous once you are pregnant, and no alternative job can be found for you, your employer must suspend you on full pay until it is safe for you to return (which may be after your maternity leave). You cannot be legally dismissed because of your pregnancy.

Male fertility and the environment

In the last few years there has been a number of newspaper headlines suggesting that if sperm counts continue to fall, mankind may become an endangered species by the year 2050. This may seem alarmist, but the fact is that, since the 1940s, the average sperm count has fallen by half. Adding to this worldwide phenomenon has been a threefold increase in testicular cancer and a twofold increase in male genital developmental abnormalities, such as undescended testes and hypospadias (where the penis is not completely formed). These developments have been so rapid in evolutionary terms that environmental factors, rather than genetic changes, are likely to be responsible.

There is a variety of possible reasons for this trend in decreasing male fertility. One is that our environment is becoming increasingly polluted with synthetic chemicals that contain oestrogen-like compounds. These have an oestrogenic effect – that is, they tend to feminize male embryos and decrease spermatogenesis (the production of sperm cells: see page 21). Many pesticides, plasticisers and detergents have an oestrogenic effect and there are traces of these in a variety of foods. Dairy cattle are sometimes given synthetic growth hormones and, as a result, the milk we drink often contains oestrogen-like compounds. Organic produce and traditionally reared meats thus make a safer choice.

Foods based on soya are also sources of phytoestrogens – oestrogen-like chemicals found naturally in many plants. Although these may have health benefits, phytoestrogens may be adding to the sum total of oestrogen-like chemicals we are exposed to. It is also possible that female hormones such as oestrogen may reach the water supply because so many women use the contraceptive pill and then excrete its by-products in their urine. However, this is unlikely to have significant effects on reproductive health.

It has been suggested that male foetuses are exposed to higher oestrogen levels in utero than previously, which may lead to poorly developed testes and male reproductive organs. Mothers today have typically low-fibre diets and this usually results in the large bowel being emptied more slowly. This means that there is more time for oestrogen to be reabsorbed and recirculated around the body. Eating a high-fibre diet that includes plenty of fruits and vegetables and wholegrain cereals will also help to reduce the reabsorption of many toxins.

In addition to these factors, men have to contend with stress, lack of exercise and increased exposure to heat, which may also contribute to lowered sperm counts.

Safeguarding your fertility against environmental hazards

There are a number of simple, practical steps you can take to reduce the risks of any pollutants and other occupational or environmental hazards affecting your fertility or unborn baby.

- When tending your garden, use organic methods. Check the labels on any products you buy to ensure they are non-toxic and safe for use during the preconception period and pregnancy.
- Complete any "do-it-yourself" home mainte-nance job involving dangerous chemicals before you conceive.
- Get your water supply checked out, and install a water filter or replace any old lead pipes if neces-sary.
- Have a risk assessment carried out at work and carry out any relevant safety measures.
- Plan ahead so that if you need any x-rays or

dental treatment involving amalgams, you can have these done before you get pregnant.
- Whenever possible, try to reduce your exposure to polluted air.
- When you shop consider buying organic food products (especially meats, fruits and vegetables), and choose non-chlorine bleached products and "green" cleaning materials.
- Consider having your home checked for radon radiation levels.

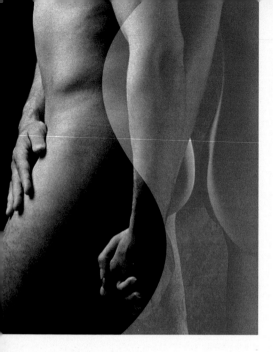

Considering Your General Health

Now that you are thinking of having a baby, you may be wondering whether any health problems you have, or have experienced in the past, will affect your chances. The impact of many common gynaecological and long-term health problems on your fertility and future pregnancies is described in this chapter. Happily, advances in medical science mean that many conditions no longer cause the insurmountable fertility problems they used to.

Gynaecological problems

If you have suffered from any gynaecological problem in the past, you may be anxious about your ability to conceive and carry a pregnancy successfully. Your doctor will be able to advise you whether your problem is likely to affect your fertility, but understanding your condition and finding suitable treatments for it are among the many positive steps you can take to improve your health and chances of conception.

Endometriosis

This very common condition causes small deposits of the endometrial tissue lining the uterus to lodge in the ovaries, Fallopian tubes, abdominal cavity and other organs close to the pelvis. The seedlings of endometrium probably travel up the Fallopian tubes during a menstrual period, where they settle outside the uterus. The trouble starts when these deposits grow and bleed in response to the normal hormonal changes that take place each month, causing pelvic pain and backache, especially during menstruation and at ovulation. As the endometrial tissue bleeds, the resulting inflammation causes scarring around the uterus, ovaries and Fallopian

tubes, and blood-filled cysts may form in the ovaries. The cysts and scarring probably lower a woman's fertility by interfering with the ovum's smooth passage from the surface of the ovary into the Fallopian tube, ready to be fertilised.

Endometriosis can affect women of any age although women who take the combined oral contraceptive pill or who begin their pregnancies in their teens or early 20s seem to be partly protected. This may be why endometriosis often emerges when a woman is in her 30s or 40s.

The effects on your fertility Severe endometriosis can lead to fertility problems by damaging the ovaries and the Fallopian tubes. However, a mild case of endometriosis is unlikely to be a fertility risk, at least while it remains mild. Many women have endometriosis without any ill effects and it is often detected coincidentally – for example, during a sterilisation operation. About seven in ten women with endometriosis don't have fertility problems. Those who suffer from pain during intercourse due to endometriosis may be less likely to conceive, simply because they avoid intercourse around the time of ovulation when their pain is at its most severe.

Treatment Endometriosis improves, often dramatically, during pregnancy and after the menopause because ovulation stops during these times and the endometriosis shrinks or even "burns out." Breast-feeding fully (see page 50) can prolong a remission after pregnancy because it inhibits ovulation and so helps to prevent the effects of endometriosis.

Medical treatment includes progestagens, danazol (a testosterone-like drug), and other drugs that stop ovulation. Because many of these drugs, especially danazol, can cause birth defects, it is vital to use a reliable contraceptive while taking them. The combined oral contraceptive pill, taken without a break, may even help in mild cases of endometriosis. However, there is no strong evidence to suggest that these treatments ultimately improve the chance of a woman becoming pregnant. Relief from the symptoms may only be temporary and the condition can return. If you are planning a family you should first discuss the benefits of each drug with your doctor – there may also be a delay in regular ovulation after the treatment finishes.

If endometriosis is thought to be causing infertility because of scarring or blockage of the delicate Fallopian tubes (viewing the abdominal cavity with a laparoscope will confirm the diagnosis), then laser treatment or microsurgery may restore a woman's fertility. Drugs may be recommended to shrink the endometriosis before surgery. Sometimes, however, a full hysterectomy is required to clear all the painful, affected tissue.

Ovarian cysts

These harmless, fluid-filled cysts found in or on the ovaries are very common and often disappear on their own. Unless they are big enough to cause a mechanical problem, they don't need to be surgically drained before you plan a pregnancy. As many as one in five women have dozens of these tiny cysts in their ovaries and a woman with these cysts is no more likely to suffer from infertility than another woman.

Natural ways to beat endometriosis

Since the role of conventional medicine in restoring fertility for endometriosis is debatable, many sufferers turn to complementary therapies for help. Most alternative practitioners take a holistic approach and address not only the endometriosis and pain it causes, but will also help you to improve your diet and adopt a healthier lifestyle.

One theory suggests that endometriosis develops in women whose immune systems are too weak to mop up the stray endometrial tissue that lodges into the abdominal cavity during menstruation. Foods that contain vitamins A, B complex, C and E, and the mineral selenium are known to help the immune system. Good, natural sources of all these vitamins and minerals can be found in the chart on pages 92–95. Some women have found a macrobiotic diet – only organically grown, mostly raw, vegetarian and vitamin-rich foods – helpful.

A hot bath with a soothing essential oil will help to ease pain associated with endometriosis, as will drinking herbal teas. If you plan to use herbal medicines, consult a medical herbalist because many herbs should be avoided during the time of preconception and pregnancy. Safe herbal teas to help relieve pain include powdered or root ginger tea (sweetened with honey), meadowsweet tea taken without milk, camomile and peppermint tea.

Polycystic ovarian syndrome (PCOS)

PCOS is less common than benign ovarian cysts. PCOS causes an imbalance of hormones. Instead of rupturing to release an ovum, ovarian follicles continue to fill with fluid, forming cysts. The ovaries continue to produce oestrogen and testosterone, which may result in increased body hair and acne. Many women with PCOS are overweight and this may be part of the problem.

The effects on your fertility Despite the pituitary's efforts to pour out luteinising hormone, the ovaries seem reluctant to release any ova, which reduces fertility. Women with PCOS usually have infrequent or irregular periods. They may be more likely to miscarry than other women.

Treatment There is no cure for PCOS but you can increase your chances of conception by trying to conceive sooner rather than later, as the ovaries become less active with age. A few women with severe PCOS will have cystic change that damages their ovaries over time, again decreasing fertility. The combined oral contraceptive pill may help to preserve the

This coloured scanning electron micrograph (SEM) shows a harmless ovarian cyst inside a human ovary. The cyst is seen on the right, coloured pink.

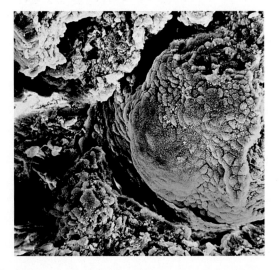

ovaries by reducing the cyst formation. If you have PCOS and are overweight, your symptoms and general health will improve with weight loss. If you have early PCOS, try to keep your weight in the ideal range (see page 101) as you will be less likely to suffer from the hormonal and metabolic effects of this syndrome later on.

Pelvic inflammatory disease (PID)

This usually occurs as a result of a sexually transmitted disease (STD), although it can also result from infections in nearby areas such as the appendix or bowel. In rare circumstances, it may occur after miscarriage, a termination or childbirth, especially if it is by caesarean section.

The symptoms of a severe attack of PID are usually pelvic pain, vaginal discharge and a fever. However, PID can often be more silent and may only cause mild abdominal pain, pain or bleeding during intercourse, or prolonged periods. Sometimes there can be no symptoms at all.

The effects on your fertility Infection or disease of the pelvic organs is a serious threat to female fertility. PID causes the uterus, ovaries and Fallopian tubes to become red, swollen and inflamed. Eventually, as the infection subsides, these organs become scarred and the Fallopian tubes can become blocked or distorted. This makes fertilisation unlikely, if not impossible. Even if the Fallopian tubes are merely distorted, a fertilised ovum may have difficulty travelling to the uterus and an ectopic pregnancy can result.

Treatment Because of its serious effects on fertility, PID should be treated urgently and any woman who has symptoms of PID should go to her doctor immediately. Antibiotics can be prescribed to treat the infection but will not reverse any scarring that has already taken place, so the earlier antibiotics are taken the less damage the disease will cause. If you catch an STD, make sure both you and your partner see a physician (see page 162) for immediate treatment.

Cervical cancer or pre-cancer

When you have a cervical smear (also known as a pap smear), a sample of cells is taken from your cervix and checked for any abnormalities which may indicate a cancer is developing. If there are any changes in these cervical cells, they are monitored carefully with further smears at more frequent intervals. If pre-cancerous cells are detected, they can be treated or removed to prevent cancer from developing.

The effects on your fertility If you have had an abnormal smear you may be wondering whether it will affect your fertility, or if having a baby will affect your cervix. Generally, the outlook is very good. If you have had abnormal cells detected or even surgical treatment for cervical cancer, your fertility is not likely to be affected. And once you become pregnant your risk of miscarriage does not increase.

If you are having frequent smears or are currently undergoing treatment for pre-cancerous or cancerous cells, you should talk to your gynaecologist who will help you choose the safest time for you to conceive. It is usually best to wait until any treatment is completed, but if you are only having follow-up smears, have one before you conceive and then again at your postnatal check-up. Smears can be taken during pregnancy but the hormonal changes that take place don't make them easy to interpret. If you think you might be pregnant when you have your cancer test, you should tell your doctor.

Treatment Early cancerous changes are treated by surgically removing some of the cervical tissue (see also page 51). Sometimes surgical excision or laser treatment is used to destroy the affected tissue. The cervix should then heal with healthy tissue and regular smears are performed to ensure this is so.

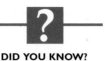

Cystitis

This very common infection or irritation of the bladder results in an urgent desire to urinate frequently, regardless of whether your bladder is full. Passing urine is usually painful and the urine may be cloudy or even contain blood. You may feel discomfort after passing urine or have abdominal pain. It is important to treat cystitis as soon as it is detected, otherwise it can lead to kidney infection and possibly cause permanent kidney damage. Women seem to be more at risk of getting cystitis than men because their urethras are much shorter and therefore more vulnerable to irritation and infection.

The effects on your fertility Cystitis should present no obstacle to your chances of conception – apart from the fact that you should abstain from intercourse until the infection has cleared up. However, it is particularly common in pregnancy because the expanding uterus places more pressure on your urethra, making it more difficult to completely empty your bladder. Increased amounts of progesterone in your body during pregnancy also make the urethra more lax, and this allows infections to travel up the urethra to the bladder more easily. If left untreated, cystitis can cause premature labour.

Treatment If a urine test shows you have cystitis, you will most likely be prescribed a course of antibiotics to treat the bacterial infection effectively. If you are planning to conceive, check with your doctor that these are safe. You can also try the natural remedies suggested in the box overleaf.

Candidiasis (yeast infection)

Also called thrush, this common infection affects many women whether they are sexually active or not. Candida is a yeast that is commonly present in the bowel and vagina, and less commonly inside the mouth. Problems arise if the yeast multiplies, especially in the vagina where it causes a white and sometimes lumpy discharge, as well as intense itching or burning. The soreness in the vaginal region makes intercourse painful and can give the same symptoms as cystitis, although it is unusual for the yeast to invade the bladder. Candida thrives well in damp places, especially if the skin is broken or sugar levels in the blood are high.

DID YOU KNOW?

Many women get cystitis when they first become sexually active or after frequent sexual intercourse. This is because when the penis is inside the vagina it can irritate the urethra, which lies next to the vagina. This is what first gave the condition in young women the name of "honeymoon cystitis."

Normally, a healthy bacteria called lactobacillus is present in the vagina which keeps the unwelcome candida at bay. However, if the balance between these is upset, thrush may develop. This can happen after taking antibiotics, which may destroy many of the normal bacteria, as well as unhealthy bacteria, and this allows candida to multiply. Women with diabetes often develop thrush because of the high sugar levels in their urine and vaginal secretions. This may also be why some women are prone to thrush after consuming a lot of sweet foods or alcoholic drinks.

Self-help measures to prevent and cure cystitis

The following will help to prevent cystitis:
- Drink lots of water, herbal teas and other clear fluids.
- Drink unsweetened cranberry juice (it has a natural antibiotic effect).
- Always completely empty your bladder – infections develop more easily in urine that becomes concentrated or stagnant. Empty your bladder before intercourse and again afterwards.
- Try to avoid vaginal deodorants, douches, bubble baths and perfumed soaps as these all irritate the urethra.
- Wear loose clothes and cotton-lined underwear to help prevent irritations and infections in the vaginal area.
- If you are using a diaphragm, make sure it fits properly or change to a cervical cap, which fits snugly over the cervix and does not press on the urethra.
- If you suffer from vaginal dryness use some lubrication.

- When you breast-feed, your body secretes protective carbohydrates, known as oligosaccharides, in both your breast milk and urine. Oligosaccharides prevent bacteria from sticking to the wall of your bladder and that of your baby's. This will protect you both from cystitis – another benefit to breast-feeding your baby.

The following will help to cure an attack of cystitis:
- As soon as symptoms start, drink at least a pint of water with a teaspoon of sodium bicarbonate (baking soda) dissolved in it. This may help to prevent any bacteria from reproducing. Continue to drink a pint of this mixture every hour until symptoms stop.
- Use a hot water bottle to relieve the pain.
- Drink unsweetened cranberry juice, hot yarrow tea and vegetable broth containing barley. These all help to ward off infection.

The effects on your fertility Although candidiasis will probably not affect your fertility, it is important to clear up any infection during pregnancy, as your baby may catch the infection from the birth canal during delivery. A baby born with candidiasis can develop nappy rash and a sore mouth, which may lead to feeding difficulties. Thrush is very common in pregnancy (affecting about one in four women) because a pregnant woman's vaginal secretions favour the growth of yeast. Men may get soreness or itching of the penis from candida but are often not affected. As candida is not sexually transmitted, your partner will only need treatment if you are having problems with recurrent thrush or if he has discomfort.

Treatment Modern antifungal treatments are usually very effective at curing an attack of thrush. Most antifungals, such as clotrimazole, can be given as a pessary and are safe during the preconception period. New oral antifungals are now available, but these are often not necessary, and as a rule they should be avoided in pregnancy because they have not been proven to be safe for the baby. An antifungal cream may help your symptoms for a few days but it will not get rid of the large reservoir of yeast present in the vagina. Lactobacillus is present in live yogurt, so for immediate treatment, try soaking a tampon in live yogurt and inserting one into your vagina twice a day for a few days. An experiment showed that women who ate 225 gm (8 ounces) of live yogurt a day reduced their risk of getting the infection by two-thirds.

Garlic has also been shown to help prevent thrush in babies and women. It can be inserted into the vagina of a woman, although it may be more effective if taken orally. You can take garlic capsules or eat it fresh, but capsules are less odorous! Allicin is the active ingredient and is also present in onions.

Candida likes a moist, warm place to grow so avoid wearing tight jeans, synthetic underwear

BACTERIAL VAGINOSIS

Also called Gardnerella vaginosis, this vaginal infection is caused by an overgrowth of vaginal bacteria. It causes an unpleasant, fishy-smelling, gray-coloured discharge, which is more noticeable after you have had sexual intercourse. Although it is usually sexually transmitted, bacterial vaginosis can be a problem in women who are not sexually active. It does not cause infertility but it may affect the quality of your cervical mucus, so it is best treated with a short course of antibiotics, such as metronidazole, before you try to conceive.

or panty liners unnecessarily. It also grows well in damaged skin so it's best to refrain from using perfumed soap, bubble bath, vaginal deodorant and douches. You should also try to limit your intake of very sweet foods and drinks, including alcohol.

Problems in previous pregnancies

If you have already had a pregnancy but suffered from a problem such as miscarriage, ectopic pregnancy or pre-eclampsia, you may be concerned about its effects on your fertility or the problem recurring in your next pregnancy. Usually the outlook is good but you may like to discuss your individual situation with your doctor before you try to conceive.

Ectopic pregnancy

The early signs of an ectopic pregnancy (one that grows outside the uterus, usually in the Fallopian tube) are abdominal pain and vaginal bleeding. As the Fallopian tube is not designed to expand, a growing embryo can rupture it, causing serious internal bleeding – a life-threatening situation for both mother and baby. An ectopic pregnancy diagnosed later than 6 weeks usually has to be treated surgically by removing the developing embryo, which almost certainly could not survive outside the uterus. Very occasionally, the embryo can be gently "milked" down the Fallopian tube and the tube is saved. When the tube is damaged it has to be surgically removed. The other tube and ovary can be checked at this time to give a woman some idea of her chance for future pregnancies.

Women at risk of having an ectopic pregnancy are those who have had one before or have had a pelvic infection caused by an STD, appendicitis, childbirth, or an operation that has damaged their Fallopian tubes, particularly a reversal of sterilisation. Endometriosis sufferers are also at increased risk. If you have already had an ectopic pregnancy or think you are at risk of having one, seek medical advice as soon as you think you might be pregnant. An ultrasound scan can confirm where the embryo is.

Miscarriage

Although miscarriage is defined as loss of a pregnancy up to 24 weeks, most miscarriages usually occur in the first four months. Some miscarriages, especially those later than six weeks, can cause heavy, painful bleeding and often a minor operation such as a D and C (dilatation and curettage) or ERPC (evacuation of retained products of conception) is needed to clear out the uterus properly and speed recovery.

Miscarriage is a difficult experience that may leave a woman feeling bereft, angry, depressed, lonely and possibly guilty. But most women go on to have a healthy pregnancy after a miscarriage, so the outlook is good, especially if you make positive changes to your diet, lifestyle and general health.

There are many myths about what causes miscarriage. Usually it occurs as a result of genetic abnormalities and is highly unlikely to be triggered by any activity the mother may engage in. The following activities do not cause miscarriage: sex in early pregnancy; exercise in early pregnancy; having a gentle internal examination or a cervical smear test; strenuous activities such as spring cleaning or decorating; or taking aspirin during a cold.

Recurrent miscarriage If you have suffered from several miscarriages there is a possibility that you or your partner may carry a genetic disorder that is affecting your chances of a successful pregnancy and you could discuss genetic counselling with your doctor (see page 65). Certain infections, including rubella (see page 168), toxoplasmosis (see page 99), and some other forms of food poisoning can also cause miscarriage, but these are unlikely to cause any future problem once the infection is over. Some animals, including cattle and sheep during lambing, can pass on a form of chlamydia (page 160) that causes miscarriage. In rare cases, structural abnormalities of the uterus, such as fibroids, may lead to miscarriage. In these instances surgery may improve a woman's chance of a successful pregnancy. If a woman has a weak or incompetent cervix that cannot hold the pregnancy until full term, her cervix can be stitched closed until it is time for the birth.

Rhesus incompatibility

Everybody has a specific blood group (A, B, AB or O) and is either Rhesus (Rh) positive or negative. Rh negative mothers who have Rh positive babies may become sensitized to the blood group cells from their babies during pregnancy and produce antibodies (proteins that defend the body from infection). These antibodies can pass into their babies' blood and destroy the babies' blood cells, resulting in anaemia. A mother is usually only sensitized at her baby's birth or if the blood cells travel into her bloodstream during a haemorrhage or miscarriage. Therefore, being Rh incompatible with a baby only becomes a problem in a second or subsequent pregnancy.

An Rh negative mother can be given an immunoglobulin injection called anti factor D to neutralise the Rh positive blood cells of her baby. This is performed within 72 hours of birth or a miscarriage. Once a mother has been treated she will not develop Rh antibodies and her next baby will be protected. If you are Rh negative, ask about the procedure at your hospital. If you don't know your blood type, make sure you get it checked to find out.

Pre-eclampsia

Some pregnant women develop raised blood pressure, and although this alone is usually not dangerous, it may be a sign that pre-eclampsia is developing. This serious condition threatens the safety of both the mother and her baby. The chief cause is probably an inadequate blood supply in the placenta, which then sends signals to the mother's circulation to raise blood pressure in an attempt to improve blood flow. The mother's kidneys are then strained and may start to leak protein. She may get swelling, called edema (swelling alone in pregnancy is common and usually harmless), and suffer from dizziness or headaches. If pre-eclampsia is not treated it can lead to life-threatening kidney or liver damage and convulsions in the mother. The baby may not grow properly because of poor placental blood supply, which is why pregnant women with pre-eclampsia are advised to take plenty of rest. If you have suffered from pre-eclampsia (or even just raised blood pressure) in a previous pregnancy you may be at increased risk, although usually less severely. There may also be an inherited risk, so if your mother or sister has suffered from pre-eclampsia make sure you get regular prenatal checks. Before you become pregnant again try to get fit to improve your circulation and start an optimum diet. In future pregnancies your doctor may also prescribe low doses of aspirin, which is one of the few drugs shown to help reduce the risk of pre-eclampsia.

Termination of pregnancy

This surgical operation is not likely to affect your future fertility unless there are complications afterwards, such as an infection. To minimise any risks to fertility, a termination should be performed in early pregnancy by a trained surgeon. Tests for possible infection should also be conducted before the operation and any infection should be treated with antibiotics to cover the time of the operation. Emotional trauma is a more real risk and if you think you would benefit from counselling before starting out on a planned pregnancy, talk to your doctor about post-termination counselling.

Minimising the risk of miscarriage

Contrary to popular belief, miscarriage rarely occurs as a result of any maternal activity. However, there are a number of steps you can take before and during pregnancy to improve your health and reduce your chances of having a miscarriage:

- Make sure you are not underweight (see page 101).
- Quit smoking – and that goes for your partner too.
- Cut down alcohol to one drink a day or less.
- Give yourselves time to recover after a miscarriage before trying to conceive again (see page 55).
- Have a health check-up (see page 169).
- Take regular and gentle exercise.
- Make sure to include all the vitamins and minerals you need in your diet.
- Tackle any stress or emotional problems in your life (see chapter 7).

Sexually transmitted diseases

These are caused by a variety of bacteria, viruses and fungi that can only be caught by sexual or intimate contact with an infected person. Some STDs have obvious symptoms but others don't, and if you or your partner has had another sexual partner, you may be at risk of carrying one. Some STDs can affect fertility by infecting semen, disrupting cervical mucus and causing serious damage – even infertility – if PID (pelvic inflammatory disease) is caused. Because babies can catch many infections during pregnancy or birth, it is vital that you have a check-up for STDs and complete any necessary treatment before you try to conceive.

Chlamydia

This infection has become the most common cause of pelvic inflammatory disease in the Western world. Chlamydia infection may be symptomless in men and women the whole time that it is causing damage, but there may be some tell-tale signs. Women with chlamydia may have increased or altered vaginal discharge and get a cervical infection that can spread up into the rest of the pelvic organs. In men especially, chlamydia can cause symptoms of urethritis.

The effects on your fertility Chlamydia can influence a woman's ability to conceive in two ways: it can lead to PID, which is a common cause of infertility and/or result in cervicitis (inflammation of the cervix), which can lead to temporary infertility by affecting the cervical mucus. Men with chlamydia may also have an infection in the testes and epididymis, which can decrease the quality of their semen. The main danger for men with chlamydia, however, is that they will pass it onto their partners who then may develop PID.

If you have a chlamydia infection and are planning a pregnancy, make sure you are treated before you conceive – a pregnant woman who has chlamydia can pass it onto her baby during birth, and the baby can suffer severe conjunctivitis and lung infections as a result.

Treatment Chlamydia is treated with the antibiotic tetracycline. Most people do not become immune to chlamydia so it is quite possible to become reinfected with the disease by another sexual partner. Because tests for chlamydia are not 100 per cent foolproof, partners should always be treated for the infection, even if their own screening test appears negative.

Gonorrhoea

Men infected by this disease nearly always suffer from a penile discharge and/or urethritis (an infection of the urethra). Women with gonorrhoea may not notice any symptoms, but a yellow vaginal discharge, cervicitis and urethral infections are all common.

The effects on your fertility If untreated, gonorrhoea in men can spread to all male sex organs and affect fertility. In women it can cause severe PID by spreading up through the cervix and infecting the uterus and Fallopian tubes, which may lead to infertility. It can also spread to the eyes, joints and throat. An infected woman can pass the bacterium on to her baby during childbirth, who may suffer from sight-threatening conjunctivitis.

Putting your feet up and getting plenty of rest may help to keep your blood pressure healthy.

Once gonorrhoea has been treated there should be no threat to your future baby.

Treatment Penicillin-related antibiotics are used to treat gonorrhoea but since other infections, such as chlamydia, are often present as well, a combination of medications may be prescribed. Treatment lasts between one and two weeks.

Syphilis

This is caused by the bacterium Treponema pallidum and is not currently common in the UK or US. Initially, syphilis causes skin rashes and ulcers but, if left untreated, it develops into a generalised illness that may remit and relapse for years. Untreated syphilis can eventually affect most parts of the body and cause permanent damage to the nervous system, including the brain.

The effects on your fertility Syphilis might not have any direct effect on your fertility, but it can be passed on to your baby during pregnancy. Babies born to mothers with syphilis tend to be small and do not thrive well; they may have birth defects of the bones, eyes, ears and teeth, and suffer from blood disorders. Therefore, to protect your baby's health, it is vital that you are treated for syphilis before you plan to conceive.

Treatment In the early stages, syphilis is treated with penicillin or other antibiotics. Because the damage caused by syphilis to the body cannot be reversed, it's vital that any suspect symptoms are checked out right away. A full genito-urinary checkup will always test for syphilis. It also tends to be routinely tested for during pregnancy.

Trichomoniasis

This is caused by an organism called Trichomon

vaginalis. Men with trichomoniasis are often symptom-free, although they can suffer from a sore glans (the tip of the penis) and urethritis. Women with trichomoniasis, however, experience an unpleasant green vaginal discharge that causes vaginal and vulval soreness.

The effects on your fertility Trichomoniasis tends not to cause pelvic infection in women, but it may interfere with the quality of the cervical mucus and this can affect fertility. Once cured, a previous attack will not affect your fertility, but make sure your partner is also infection-free.

Treatment A course of metronidazole is usually prescribed to clear up the condition. Alcohol should be avoided while taking this drug.

Genital herpes

Caused by the herpes simplex virus, this STD causes tiny, painful ulcers around the vagina and cervix in women, and on the penis in men. Once a person has been infected by the herpes virus, the infection may be life-long; the virus lies dormant in the nerve cells and flares up during times of stress or illness, although there may be months or years between attacks. Usually, herpes can only be transmitted to your partner when you have an attack of the herpes infection, with ulcers and blisters.

The effects on your fertility Having herpes will not affect your ability to conceive, and does not tend to affect a baby even during pregnancy. However, an attack (especially a first infection) near the time of birth could result in the baby catching the infection during delivery, causing serious illness. If a mother has an episode of herpes at the end of her pregnancy, a caesarean section may be performed to stop the baby

Recognising the symptoms of STDs

Many STDs give only minor symptoms even though they are silently causing damage to your fertility. Sometimes one partner may be affected with severe symptoms but the other is apparently unaffected. This is why both partners should always be tested and treated.

Common STD symptoms for women include abnormal vaginal discharge, cystitis, rashes around the pubic region, pain during intercourse, lower abdominal pain if the pelvic organs are affected, and a painfully swollen vulva. Common symptoms for men include discharge from the penis, soreness or ulcers, a frequent urge to urinate and pain while passing urine (urethritis), swollen glands in the groin, and painful testes or prostate gland.

If you suspect you have an STD you should consult your gynaecologist or attend a genito-urinary clinic for a check-up (see also page 162).

---

coming into contact with the virus in the vagina during birth.

Treatment Acyclovir and other antiviral drugs are helpful in shortening attacks but cannot cure the disease completely.

Genital warts

These are caused by the human papilloma virus (HPV) and can cause small, unpleasant and lumpy skin growths around the vagina, cervix, anus, or penis. Women with genital warts may be prone to cervical cancer and should have regular smears.

The effects on your fertility Although warts themselves are not a fertility risk, other infections may often be present. Anyone who suspects they have warts should have a full genito-urinary check-up (see box opposite) to ensure they haven't caught any other infection.

Treatment Genital warts can be treated by freezing or with podophyllin medication.

Human immunodeficiency virus (HIV)

HIV infection can lead to the disease known as AIDS (autoimmune deficiency syndrome). The HIV virus attacks the body's natural "killer" cells (called T-helper cells), which normally defend it from a wide range of infections and some kinds of cancer. The body's immune system is gradually worn down by the virus and the HIV sufferer may become afflicted with AIDS-related illnesses, such as life-threatening infections, skin rashes and tumours of the lymph glands.

HIV can be transmitted by sexual contact, needle sharing, blood transfusions and by pregnant mothers to their babies. The virus can only be detected about three months after it has been acquired because it takes this long for antibodies to appear in the blood. Although the body forms these antibodies, they are not able to wipe out the infection, which lies hidden inside the body's immune cells. Fifty per cent of people with HIV infection will develop AIDS within ten years.

The effects on your fertility A woman's fertility may not be affected at all by HIV or AIDS, but this potentially fatal and untreatable infection presents very serious threats to pregnancy and motherhood. Babies of mothers infected with HIV may be born with the virus and are likely to develop AIDS by their second birthday. Breast-feeding mothers with HIV can also transmit the virus to their children.

Treatment As yet, there is no cure or immunisation against HIV. However, in some cases drug combinations can help to bring remission.

Long-term medical problems

Some medical conditions have no direct impact on your fertility but they may have repercussions in pregnancy (for both you and your baby), and later in parenthood. Thankfully, medical care has improved so much over the last few decades that many of these problems can now be controlled – if not completely cured – so that women who previously would not have considered risking pregnancy are now able to go through pregnancy and childbirth safely.

Diabetes mellitus

This disorder, where the pancreas produces insufficient amounts of insulin to regulate the body's sugar and starch levels, causes high levels of sugar in the blood but starves many organs of their supply of energy, leading to excessive thirst and a high urine output. Until insulin was introduced as a treatment for diabetes in 1922, pregnancy was often fatal for the diabetic mother. Even after insulin was introduced, babies born to diabetic mothers frequently died soon after birth or had birth defects, although the mothers' health was no longer in such danger. Over the last few decades, however, doctors have shown that good pre-pregnancy care can dramatically improve the outlook for diabetic mothers-to-be and their babies.

The implications for your fertility
Pregnancy may be a risk for a diabetic woman because it may worsen any ill effects, such as raised blood pressure or kidney damage. However, if she is healthy and takes good care, pregnancy need not be dangerous.

Babies who are born to mothers with poorly controlled diabetes may suffer from two main problems. The first is a tendency to develop defects of the major organs. The good news is that the better the diabetes is controlled, the lower the risk. In fact, mothers with well-controlled diabetes before conception and in pregnancy are probably not at any greater risk of having a baby with birth defects than mothers without the condition.

Having a genito-urinary check-up

If you or your partner are at risk of having acquired an STD – even if you show no symptoms – you should attend a genito-urinary (GU) clinic for a proper check-up before you conceive. GU clinics are the best place to receive an accurate diagnosis of STDs because they have the facilities to examine swabs and microscope slides immediately and can often give you a result within days. You can find your local GU clinic in the telephone book.

At the GU clinic your attending doctor will ask you for a detailed medical history, including previous sexual partners and any pregnancies. You will then be examined. As well as a genital examination this may include a general check-up, especially if you feel unwell or have a rash. Swabs will be taken from your urethra, vagina and cervix. Unless you are bleeding, a cervical smear will also probably be taken. For men, a urethral swab will be taken and, in some cases, a specimen of semen might be required. These tests should be painless, although a little uncomfortable. Both men and women will have a sample of their urine tested. Blood tests can be used to help diagnose herpes and syphilis, but blood tests for HIV will only be taken after counselling and if you agree to it.

If you have an STD you will be offered treatment. As well as undergoing this treatment, you should also return to make sure you have been cured. Check with your doctor to see if your partner should be treated too.

The second problem is that babies whose mothers have high blood sugar levels during pregnancy tend to be rather big, but despite their size, they act as premature babies at birth. As a result of coping with the extra sugar crossing the placenta during pregnancy, these babies often tend to have high insulin levels as well. When born, they usually need special care to keep their blood sugars up to normal, and they sometimes suffer from immature lungs and breathing difficulties.

If you have diabetes the key to a healthy baby is planning your pregnancy so you keep your blood sugar levels as normal as possible from before you conceive, right through the early weeks of pregnancy – when your baby is developing all his vital organs – until the very end of your pregnancy. Well before you plan to conceive, ask your doctor for advice about monitoring your blood sugar levels more frequently and administering your insulin. Find out if your local hospital has a pre-pregnancy diabetic clinic that you can attend for regular checks and advice.

Although children of a diabetic parent are at a slightly increased risk of developing diabetes, only about 3 in 100 will do so. If both parents are diabetic the risk may be slightly higher.

Epilepsy

Having seizures or convulsions is unlikely to affect your fertility unless you are one of the few women who suffer from irregular and infrequent periods as a result of your medication, which could delay conception. During pregnancy, some women experience more convulsions, possibly as a result of the hormone changes decreasing the anticonvulsant levels in their blood. Taking blood tests to monitor these levels and adjusting medication may help. But, happily, nine out of ten women with epilepsy do not have an increase in fits during pregnancy.

The implications for your fertility The main problem for epilepsy sufferers who would like to become pregnant is that many of the anticonvulsant drugs, especially sodium valproate, phenytoin, phenobarbitone and carbamazepine can cause severe birth defects, such as heart problems, spina bifida, cleft palate, an undeveloped penis (hypospadias), and unseparated fingers. Some of the more modern drugs, including gabapentin and lamotrigine, seem to be safer but they have not been in use long enough for experts to be sure.

If you have suffered from epileptic fits or currently take anticonvulsant drugs, discuss with your doctor the impact this may have on a pregnancy before you conceive – many birth defects caused by epilepsy medication occur in the first few weeks after conception. If you do not have severe epilepsy and have been free of fits for more than a year, your doctor may consider it safe for you to stop or reduce your medication, at least for the first 12 weeks of pregnancy while

Genito-urinary clinics have all the facilities to take swabs and examine them under microscope immediately. They can usually provide a result within a few days.

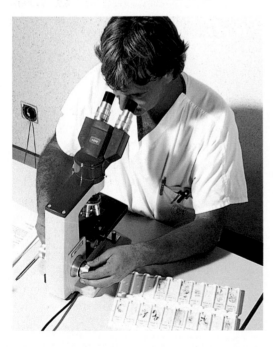

your baby's vital organs are forming. If this is not possible, he or she may change your medication to a safer drug, or divide the dose so that you take smaller amounts more frequently. This will help to avoid exposing your baby to sudden high levels of drugs. As spina bifida is a particular risk for babies exposed to sodium valproate and many other anticonvulsant drugs, epileptic mothers are advised to take a high, daily dose of folic acid (usually 4 or 5 mg) from before the time of conception, as well as during pregnancy (see also page 89).

Asthma

The effects of this reversible narrowing of the airways in the lungs vary from a slight breathlessness and wheezing to a life-threatening lack of oxygen.

The implications for your fertility
Generally, pregnancy does not seem to make asthma worse unless increased stress is already a trigger. Most mild asthma attacks are treated with inhaled medication, which does not have any impact on a developing baby. The main concern is whether long-term oral steroid medication will affect the unborn baby. Overall, there does not seem to be much evidence of an increased risk of birth defects in this case, although mothers with severe asthmatic attacks during pregnancy may have slightly smaller babies.

Asthma tends to run in families, especially when allergies are a problem. About 1 in 20 of all babies may develop asthma but the risk is trebled if one parent has asthma. If both parents are affected the risk is higher. If you suffer from asthma and you want to avoid passing it on to your child, the season in which you conceive can have an effect, as well as exposure to allergens in your baby's first few months of life (see page 67). Breast-feeding can also help.

TIME TO TALK

The implications of health problems

Future parents with a health problem will need to consider if pregnancy will be a risk to the mother's health and whether their baby will be born healthy. Some of the questions you may need to discuss with your doctor include:

- Will my condition or the medication I take affect my chance of becoming pregnant?
- Will the medication I take affect my developing baby during pregnancy?
- Can I stop my medication while I try to get pregnant or take a safe, alternative medication?
- Will pregnancy make my condition worse?
- Could my health problem be inherited?
- Will I be fit enough to cope with the demands of looking after a baby and, later, a lively toddler?
- If my condition is life-threatening, can I expect to raise my child through to adulthood?

Lupus erythematosis

This is an autoimmune disease where, for unknown reasons, the body's defence system attacks its own tissues. It causes rashes and joint pains, and, in severe cases, damages vital organs such as the kidneys. Lupus erythematosis (often shortened to lupus) affects ten times as many women as men and there seems to be a higher incidence of it among people of African, West Indian and Chinese origin.

The implications for your fertility Some women with lupus erythematosis develop antiphospholipid antibodies, and these can cause thromboses or blood clots. This is known as the antiphospholipid syndrome (APS). Women with APS may not have difficulty conceiving, but could experience recurrent miscarriages. Small blood clots form in the placenta, causing it to fail and the pregnancy to be lost. Recent research suggests that up to 20 per cent of women who

LOOKING AHEAD **Gestational diabetes**

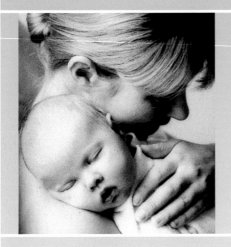

A pregnant woman may develop what is called gestational diabetes. This is different to the diabetes that requires life-long insulin treatment, as it usually lasts only during pregnancy and is not normally a serious hazard for the mother or baby.

This arises because some pregnancy hormones tend to increase the mother's blood sugar levels. Even though a woman with gestational diabetes can produce insulin (the vital hormone that regulates blood sugar levels), her body's system is overwhelmed. As a result, blood sugar spills over into her urine and high levels are also passed on to her baby. A pregnant woman's urine is usually tested for this in prenatal check-ups. If you have suffered from gestational diabetes previously, you have a one in two chance of developing it again in your next pregnancy. As it tends to occur later in pregnancy, the baby is not at high risk of developing a birth defect.

However, he may suffer from some of the effects of his mother's high glucose levels and may need special care at birth. If the condition becomes severe during pregnancy, changes in your diet will help to control it. Sugary foods will raise your blood sugar levels, so it is a good idea to cut these out of your diet. If you are overweight you may be able to reduce the risk of gestational diabetes by losing weight before you conceive (see page 103).

have suffered from three or more miscarriages may have APS.

Treatment for APS is developing fast and many sufferers are now taking low dose aspirin to help prevent blood clots and miscarriage. Heparin (an anticoagulant) can also be used but has to be given by injection, which is more inconvenient. Aspirin and heparin combined may give the best chance of a successful pregnancy for women with APS. If you are diagnosed with lupus or APS ask your doctor to refer you to a specialist with experience in this condition, who can advise and treat you in pregnancy.

Hypertension (high blood pressure)

This occurs when your blood circulates under high pressure, putting your heart and blood vessels under stress. In time, high blood pressure can cause damage to your blood vessels, especially in the kidneys, brain, and those supplying blood to the heart.

The implications for your fertility If you are one of the few young women who suffer from hypertension, you are probably taking medication. Because some antihypertensive drugs cause birth defects you should check with your doctor before you conceive to make sure any medication you take for this problem is safe. You can also refer to the chart at the end of this chapter. If you have high blood pressure, you are more likely to develop pre-eclampsia during pregnancy (see page 159) so once you have conceived, make sure you visit your doctor for frequent prenatal checks.

Kidney problems

These include a wide variety of problems, such as infection, damage and congenital defects, which can all decrease kidney function.

The implications for your fertility During pregnancy your kidneys have to work extra hard to excrete the waste produced by both you and your baby, so they enlarge to cope with the demand.

If you have kidney problems, especially if you also have high blood pressure, you may be at risk of developing pre-eclampsia, so have regular prenatal checks once you conceive. If you have had a kidney transplant, you may be able to have a successful pregnancy but you will need to consult your doctor who can assess your individual risk.

Any woman with kidney problems embarking on a pregnancy needs to take great care to avoid cystitis as this may lead to kidney infection and damage. Drink plenty of fluids throughout the day, especially when the weather is hot, and treat early signs of cystitis right away, taking a urine specimen to your doctor for testing. Since anaemia can also be a problem associated with kidney disease, you should have your blood checked before you try to conceive.

Heart disease

Although heart attacks and angina are rare in young women of childbearing age, some women hoping to become pregnant may have been born with a heart defect or may have acquired a damaged heart valve through rheumatic fever.

The implications for your fertility If you were born with a heart defect or have an acquired problem, but now live a normal life, the chances are that a pregnancy will be safe for you and your baby. Your heart does have to cope with a big increase in blood flow during pregnancy, however, and women whose lungs have begun to suffer from the effects of heart disease and get breathless, or who have poor circulation, may put themselves at serious risk by becoming pregnant. If this is your case, you should discuss the potential dangers with your doctor before conceiving. Your baby is only likely to suffer if your circulation is very poor and cannot nourish the placenta properly.

If you are taking regular medication for heart disease you should seek medical advice

---

MULTIPLE SCLEROSIS (MS)

The most common neurological disease to affect young adults in the UK, multiple sclerosis (MS) afflicts more women than men. MS does not affect female fertility, but male sufferers could experience erectile difficulties, making it hard to conceive.

In the past, women with MS were counselled to avoid pregnancy for fear it would cause a serious deterioration in their condition. Thankfully, research has now shown that although women with MS have a one in four chance of suffering a relapse after delivery, this does not cause a long-term worsening of their symptoms. In fact, many women feel better than ever during pregnancy.

Sufferers hoping to start a family should plan ahead and check with their doctor that the drugs they are taking are safe. They should also include plenty of essential fatty acids in their diet as these are vital for nerve function. To decrease the risk of relapse after birth, women should arrange for plenty of help so they can rest properly. They should also seek immediate treatment for any infections.

Difficult diagnosis, simple treatment

Marion, a lawyer, was twenty-five years old and working in a busy law practice when she first miscarried after 13 weeks of pregnancy. At the time, she was reassured by her doctor that miscarriage was a common occurrence and was told not to worry about it. But after two more miscarriages in just as many years, Marion was beginning to get a desperate feeling that she would never have a baby.

"After my third miscarriage, I got really disheartened and went to see my doctor again for more advice. My doctor asked me some detailed questions, one of which was whether I had any rashes. It did occur to me that I often noticed a mild rash on my face. I had also recently started getting the odd joint pain. I hadn't really thought much of these symptoms, having just put them down to the stressful life I was leading at the time. When I mentioned the rashes to my

doctor, she referred me to a gynaecologist who tested me for autoimmune diseases.

When the results came back, my doctor told me I had high levels of antiphospholipid antibodies and was suffering from a mild form of lupus. I had never heard of this, so was surprised to learn it was very common. I was prescribed a low, daily dose of aspirin, which didn't interfere with my life too much, and soon after I started the medication, I conceived again. Obviously, I was terrified I'd lose the baby again, so I went to see my doctor for prenatal advice. She said I could take more medication in the form of heparin injections, but an ultrasound showed that my baby was growing well, so I decided not to. My pregnancy progressed really smoothly – I didn't even get much morning sickness! – and after 37 weeks, I was overjoyed when I gave birth to a healthy baby boy."

before you attempt to conceive. If you are using warfarin to prevent thrombosis, your doctor will probably change your medication to injections of heparin, at least for the first three months of your pregnancy, as it is known to be safer for the baby. If you have a congenital heart disease, you should also seek genetic counselling (see page 65) to assess any possible risk of your baby being born with a heart problem too.

Cystic fibrosis

This is a life-threatening inherited disease in which the body's secretions are thickened, causing severe damage to the lungs and the digestive system. Before effective treatments were available, most sufferers died in childhood. But now that physiotherapy and drug treatment for cystic fibrosis are so effective, young men and women frequently survive into adulthood and a few women consider having a family (most men with cystic fibrosis are infertile as the vas deferens does not develop properly).

The implications for your fertility Future parents with cystic fibrosis do have to face the reality that their life expectancy is only 30 to 40 years on average, and women who are severely affected may be advised by the doctor that a pregnancy could be a serious risk to their health.

About 1 in 20 people in the UK and 1 in 20 in the US carry the gene for cystic fibrosis. If both parents carry the gene (even though they are not affected) then their child has a one in four chance of being affected with the disease. If a parent has cystic fibrosis then all the children will become carriers of the gene, but they will only risk inheriting the disease if the other parent is a carrier (see inherited disorders, page 66). Genetic testing on a mouthwash sample can usually pick up most carriers, so if you have a family history of cystic fibrosis or suffer from it yourself you should seek expert genetic counselling and testing before considering a pregnancy.

Cancer

Many childhood cancers, such as leukemia, were once fatal. Nowadays, many sufferers have successful treatment and survive into adulthood. Many adult cancers, such as breast and skin cancer, can now be treated and this gives men and women the chance to consider parenthood.

The implications for your fertility If you have had successful treatment for a cancer in the past, you probably have a number of questions about the effects it may have had on your fertility, especially if you have since been given the "all clear." Unless your treatment involved radiation of the pelvis, in which case your fertility may have been damaged, the evidence seems to be reassuring. A recent Canadian study indicated that parents of children born with birth defects were no more likely to have had cancer treatment than other parents whose children were born without defects.

Previously, women who had treatment for breast cancer were thought to have an increased risk of further cancer if they became pregnant. This is no longer thought to be the case. Of

VACCINATIONS

Some viral illnesses, such as rubella (German measles) and toxoplasmosis (a food-borne infection: see also page 98), can cause severe damage to your unborn baby if you catch them while you are pregnant. You will probably have already been immunised against all the common childhood viral illnesses, such as rubella, measles, mumps, or polio, or you may have become immune naturally. However, it is worth taking a blood test before you plan to conceive to confirm your immunity.

If you need to be immunised against rubella, or need a vaccination before travelling abroad or starting a new job, make sure you use effective contraception so you don't become pregnant in the next three months. This is because many vaccines, including rubella and polio, contain live viruses that could harm a growing baby. If you or your partner have had a viral infection, such as flu or glandular fever, wait until you feel better – a sign that your body has overcome the infection – before trying to conceive.

Your preconception check-up

Before you start thinking about getting pregnant, it's best to get a clean bill of health from your doctor. Your preconception check-up should include the following:

- Checking your immune status, especially against rubella and toxoplasmosis.
- Attending a GU clinic if you think you are at risk of having an STD.
- Having a urine test to check for infection and glucose.
- Getting your blood pressure taken.
- Having a cervical smear if you have not had one in recent months.
- Testing your blood group to discover whether you are Rhesus negative.
- Discussing with your doctor the implications of any long-term health problem for fertility, pregnancy and parenthood.
- Making sure any medication you take is safe during pregnancy and will not affect your fertility.

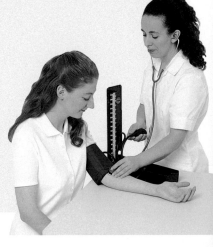

course, if you have had any form of cancer diagnosed in the past, especially if you have recently undergone treatment, you will still need to face the serious question of whether your health is up to the long and demanding challenges that parenthood poses. In order to do this, you will need to take the time to sit down and discuss your own particular circumstances with both your partner and your doctor.

Thyroid problems

The thyroid gland is situated at the front of the neck and is important for regulating the body's metabolic rate. If her thyroid is underactive or overactive, a woman can experience menstrual problems, infertility or miscarriage.

The implications for your fertility If you have a thyroid problem that is stable and being effectively treated, then your fertility is not likely to be affected. Carbimazole is commonly given to treat an overactive thyroid and is unlikely to cause birth defects. Thyroxine is given to compensate for an underactive thyroid and is

---

IF YOU NEED MEDICATION BEFORE AND DURING PREGNANCY

If you are taking medication, let your doctor or pharmacist know that you are planning a pregnancy, or if you think you may be pregnant already. No drug can be guaranteed safe in pregnancy and some are known to damage a developing baby. Others are best avoided in early pregnancy, but are probably safe later when the baby's organs have developed and the risk of birth defects is lower. In exceptional circumstances, some of the drugs listed here may be used under medical supervision when the risks to the mother outweigh the theoretical risks to the child. For more information, talk to your doctor.

COMMONLY USED MEDICINES THAT ARE PROBABLY SAFE IN EARLY PREGNANCY

Antacids used to treat indigestion (but you should try to avoid aluminium-based products where possible).
Anxiolytics and other sedatives taken for anxiety.

Corticosteroids used to treat asthma.
Clotrimazole and other vaginal thrush treatments.
Ephedrine used in common cold remedies.

Aspirin (except possibly in late pregnancy, but check with your doctor).
Penicillin (an antibiotic).
Cephalosporins (antibiotics).
Sodium chromoglycate used to treat hayfever and asthma.

DRUGS THAT ARE PROBABLY SAFE BUT SHOULD BE USED ONLY WHEN NECESSARY AND UPON MEDICAL ADVICE

Acyclovir used for herpes and cold sores.
Antidepressants of the monoamine oxidase inhibitor type.
Antihistamines such as chlorpheniramine, used to treat hayfever and other common allergies.

Antipsychotics used to treat psychotic disorders, such as schizophrenia.
Blood pressure medication that is not listed below.
Carbimazole used to treat an overactive thyroid.

Gamma linolenic acid used to treat PMS, particularly breast pain.
Heparin an anticoagulant used to treat thrombosis.
Sumatriptan used to treat migraine.
Tetracycline an antibiotic. (Causes discoloration of the baby's teeth so avoid in the last six months of pregnancy.)

vital for your baby's health. If you choose to breast-feed your baby, your doctor may change you on to a different drug if the existing medication you take could be passed on to your baby through breast milk.

If you are suffering from a thyroid disease your baby will be given special thyroid tests after her birth because a healthy thyroid is vital for proper brain development. This special test is in addition to the routine test given to all newborn babies to test for thyroid deficiency.

DID YOU KNOW?

If your partner has had a severe illness, such as hepatitis or glandular fever, it's important that you wait at least three months before you try to get pregnant. This is the length of time required for new, healthy sperm to form and mature.

TO BE AVOIDED AROUND CONCEPTION AND IN EARLY PREGNANCY
(EXCEPT UNDER EXPERT MEDICAL GUIDANCE)

ACE inhibitors used to treat high blood pressure and heart failure.

Acetretin, isotretinoin and all retinoid derived skin preparations taken by mouth used to treat acne and psoriasis.

Amphetamines used in dieting.

Anabolic steroids and androgens used for body building and in hormonal disorders.

Anticoagulants such as warfarin, except under medical supervision. Used to thin the blood following deep vein thrombosis and in heart conditions.

Anticonvulsants (Some are safer than others, so make sure you check with your doctor.)

Antidepressants (Except under medical direction.)

Astemizole an antihistamine.

Beta blockers used to treat hypertension and anxiety.

Carbamazepine used to treat epilepsy.

Clofibrate used to lower cholesterol.

Clotrimazole an antibiotic.

Cytotoxic drugs used in cancer treatment.

Cyproterone used to treat acne and polycystic ovarian syndrome.

Danazol used for endometriosis.

Dexamphetamine used for certain epileptic conditions.

Disulfiram used in alcohol addiction.

Diuretics used to treat fluid retention.

Ergotamine taken for migraines.

Fluconazole and ketoconazole taken orally for thrush (most topical treatments are safe).

Gold used to treat rheumatoid arthritis.

Griseofulvin an antifungal prescribed for nail infections.

Idoxuridine used for cold sores.

Radioactive iodine for treating overactive thyroid disease.

Lithium used to treat long-term depression.

Mefloquine used to prevent malaria.

Metformin used for diabetes.

Metronidazole for treatment of sexually transmitted and other vaginal infections.

Nicotine replacement therapies

Phenobarbitone used to treat epilepsy.

Piperazine, thiabendazole and other drugs used to treat worm infestation.

Podophyllum used for warts.

Progestagen hormones used to treat menstrual disorders.

Rifampin used to treat tuberculosis.

Sodium valproate used to treat epilepsy.

Tamoxifen for breast cancer and other breast disorders.

Vaccines that contain live viruses, such as rubella or polio.

YOUR QUICK REFERENCE ACTION PLAN

Plan your pregnancy

- Talk with your partner about the implications of parenthood and make sure that you are both happy to start a family.

- Allow at least three months to get fit and improve your lifestyle.

- Consider any previous or long-term health problems.

- If you had problems in a previous pregnancy, for example, pre-eclampsia, talk to your doctor.

- If you need to take medication, make sure your doctor knows you are planning to get pregnant.

- Allow sufficient time to pass since an earlier conception or pregnancy.

- See a genetic counsellor if you are worried about inherited diseases in either side of your families or you have had repeated miscarriages.

Have a medical check-up

- Have a blood test to see if you are immune to rubella and toxoplasmosis.

- Check your blood group. If you are rhesus negative, check with your doctor about treatment at birth or if you should bleed in pregnancy.

- Make sure you are not anaemic. If you are, treat this before you become pregnant.

- If you have irregular periods, check that your thyroid function is normal.

- Have a cervical smear to confirm that your cervix is healthy.

- If you have been at risk of an STD infection, visit a GU clinic for a check-up and complete any treatment before trying to conceive.

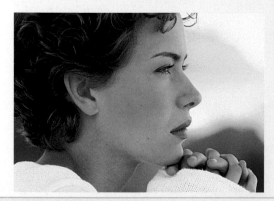
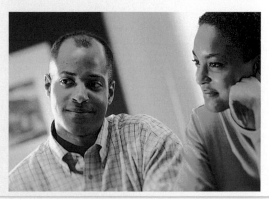

Now that you have read Parts 1 and 2 of this book, you will understand the importance of preparing yourselves for conception. Here is a summary plan to help make sure you improve your health in every area.

Boost your fertility

- Try charting your menstrual cycle to learn your fertile times. You might like to seek the advice of a fertility awareness teacher to help you on this.

- Check your method of contraception. If you are using a hormonal method of contraception, you may want to change to a barrier method or natural family planning method before you conceive.

- Improve your diet so you are getting the right amount of all the vitamins and minerals you need. You can consider vitamin supplements, especially for folic acid to prevent spina bifida.

- Take care when preparing food and dealing with animals to avoid food infections such as toxoplasmosis and listeriosis.

- Protect yourself from toxic chemicals and ionising radiation in the workplace and at home.

Get into shape

- Keep your weight in the fertile range.

- Make sure you get enough exercise.

- Learn a relaxation technique to help you counter stress and anxiety.

- Stop smoking tobacco or using nicotine replacement products.

- Cut your alcohol intake to safe levels or consider avoiding it altogether.

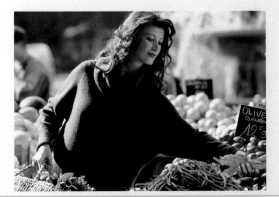

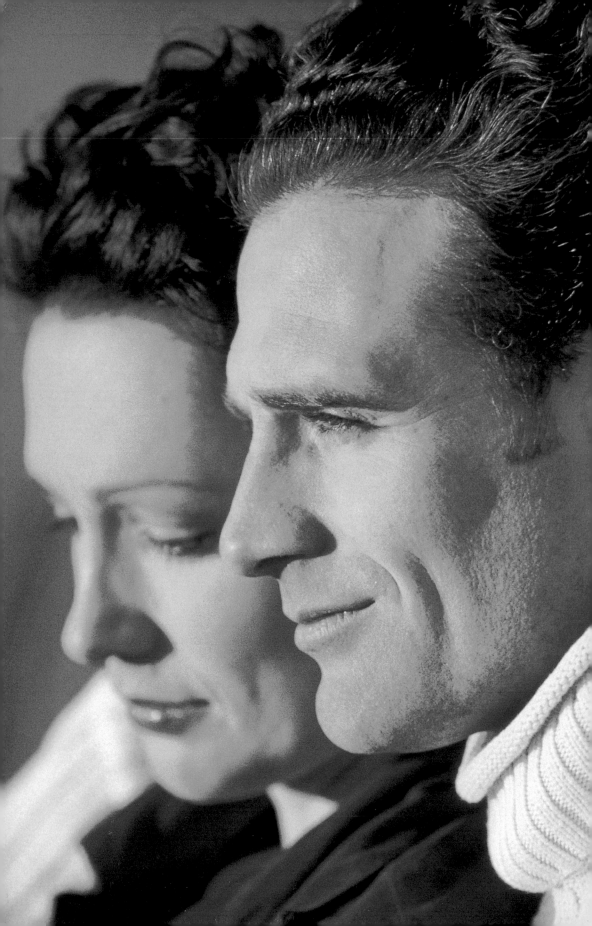

PART III

IF CONCEPTION
DOESN'T HAPPEN

For some couples pregnancy comes effortlessly, sometimes even as a bit of a surprise. Most healthy young couples will conceive naturally within two years of unprotected intercourse, but for those who don't, period follows period each month with distressing monotony. If you have made all the health improvements suggested in previous chapters and are still having difficulty conceiving, you may need medical help to investigate the cause of your difficulty in conceiving.

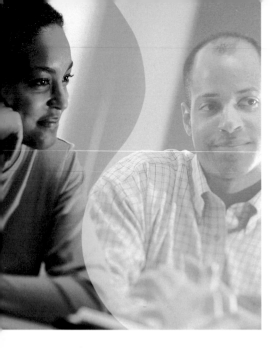

What Next?

Sometimes there is an identifiable medical reason why, after a year or two of trying, you still cannot get pregnant. This chapter looks at the most common causes of fertility problems and the help that medical science can (and can't) provide. If you do need help with conception, remember to keep yourself in good health – whether you conceive naturally or with medical assistance, your baby's health depends on yours. If you smoke or survive on a poor diet, no amount of infertility investigation or treatment will guarantee a healthy pregnancy or protect your baby from possible harm.

Investigating infertility

According to the British fertility expert, Professor Lord Robert Winston, too many couples with fertility problems are under-investigated and told there is nothing wrong. In actual fact, with thorough investigation around 96 per cent of couples with fertility problems will end up with a known cause for their difficulties. The reasons for a couple's inability to conceive are divided more or less equally into three areas: the problem may lie with the woman, the man or with both partners.

If you and your partner are both under the age of 30 and have no obvious health problems, you probably will not need fertility tests or treatment unless you have been trying to conceive unsuccessfully for two years. Most doctors agree that after the age of 30, a couple should be seen by a fertility specialist after only one year of trying. For couples where the woman is over the age of 35, a doctor might make a referral to a fertility specialist more quickly. If your periods are very infrequent or absent, you should seek advice right away.

Male fertility problems

In recent years, research into male infertility has increased and this has led to improved diagnosis and some hopeful new treatments. Experts are now recognising more causes of male fertility problems and looking for solutions to these. The main problems men experience with their fertility are due to difficulties with sexual intercourse or are caused by poor sperm quality. Now that sperm quality is known to be decreasing in many parts of the world (see also page 150) ways to combat this trend need to be found.

Poor sperm quality This is one of the main causes of male infertility. Poor sperm quality can cover a multitude of problems, including lowered sperm count, a significant proportion of abnormal sperm, and sperm that have poor motility (ability to swim forwards effectively). Many of the general health issues discussed in this book (such as smoking, drinking alcohol, taking medication, obesity, exposure to heat and chemicals) contribute to poor semen quality, but there are also other factors.

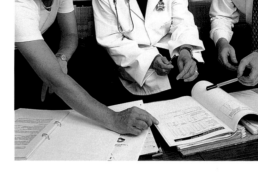

Sometimes hormonal problems prevent a man from producing enough sperm. For instance, his hypothalamus and pituitary glands may fail to send out sufficient levels of LH and FSH, the hormones that stimulate testosterone production and spermatogenesis. This can sometimes be treated with hormone replacement therapy. In some cases, despite sufficient levels of LH and FSH, the testes simply fail to respond to these hormones. Unfortunately, there is no treatment for this. Many of the general health factors that have such a detrimental effect on fertility, such as smoking and alcohol, do so by decreasing testosterone production and therefore reducing semen quality.

For the many couples whose hope for the future relies on effective and safe fertility treatment, the increasing investment in up-to-date research is good news.

Many sexually transmitted infections can reduce the motility of sperm. Infections of the prostate can reduce overall sperm count as well as motility, but sperm production usually recovers once the infection has been treated. Some viral infections, notably mumps, can infect the testes and permanently reduce sperm production. If a man catches mumps, he may be given medical treatment to help prevent testicular damage, although this is not always possible.

Varicose veins in the testes, known as varicoceles, can reduce a man's sperm count, probably by acting as a heat source. Varicoceles feel like a bag of worms in the scrotum and can usually be removed surgically or injected with a chemical solution that causes the vein to scar over and remain closed.

As many as one in ten men suffering fertility problems has antibodies to his own sperm. These may form after an injury to the groin area – when bruising and torn tissue around the scrotum and vas deferens allow sperm and blood to mix – or, more commonly, after reversal of a vasectomy.

Protein from the sperm that have entered the blood stream is recognised by a man's body as foreign because it contains different genetic material. In response to this, the man's immune system forms antibodies that attack and destroy healthy sperm, reducing motility and sometimes the sperm count. Some men have been helped by steroids to reduce this reaction but success is limited.

Some men who suffer from reduced sperm count may think that by "saving it up" and refraining from frequent intercourse, they will strengthen their sperm count. Although the sperm count may rise after a few days of abstinence, after five days of abstinence the motility of the sperm may start to suffer. Frequent ejaculation stimulates the testes and epididymides to produce fresh sperm, although men with very low sperm counts may be advised to have sex on alternate days.

Getting in shape can increase the quality of a man's sperm and improve the blood flow to his reproductive organs. This may help to prevent any erectile difficulties.

No sperm production Some men may be born with abnormalities that can affect the process of sperm manufacture. For example, boys born with undescended testes won't be able to produce sperm because the testes are not at a cool enough temperature. Boys born with blocked vasa deferensa will have no sperm in their semen. Men with cystic fibrosis may not develop a vas deferens and may have very low sperm production (which is why most men with cystic fibrosis are infertile). Rarely, a hidden chromosomal defect may account for absent or poor sperm production. Some congenital disorders, such as undescended testes, may be treated surgically.

Problems with sperm delivery Another cause of fertility difficulties for men is not being able to deposit sperm into the vagina. This may be due to retrograde ejaculation (when sperm is pumped backwards into the bladder instead of out of the penis), premature ejaculation, or erectile or ejaculatory failure.

Impotence is an emotive word covering all sorts of difficulties that men might have with erection and ejaculation. Erectile problems may have a physical cause, such as damaged nerve supply to the penis as a result of diabetes, or side effects of medication such as tranquillizers, antidepressants and diuretics. Sometimes atherosclerosis of the arteries supplying the testes and penis can cause impotence – not enough blood is being supplied to maintain an erection. Pelvic floor exercises that strengthen the muscles around the erectile tissues in the penis can help improve blood flow and erection.

More often, however, difficulties with starting or maintaining an erection are emotional and caused by stress, anger or anxiety. If you cannot achieve or maintain a satisfactory erection, but still have erections at night or on waking, the problem is most likely to be psychological (see also chapter 7: Improving Your Physical and Emotional Health). This kind of impotence can often be overcome with counselling and close cooperation and communication with your partner.

For men who sometimes ejaculate too soon before penetration (known as premature ejaculation), there are simple techniques that couples can learn to help a man delay ejaculation. These involve alternate gentle stimulation and relaxation, which enables the man to control erection and ejaculation more easily. Retrograde ejaculation can sometimes be treated by a surgical operation. Semen running out of the vagina shortly after intercourse, however, is not a cause for concern. This phenomenon, called effluvium seminis, is normal and usually happens in the hour after intercourse as the semen, which initially clots, starts to liquefy under the influence of enzymes. Plenty of healthy sperm start the journey through the cervix within minutes of ejaculation and many thousands of others will swim around in the cervical mucus at the top of the vagina for a while. As long as penetration occurs during intercourse, sperm will be able to embark on their journey to the ovum.

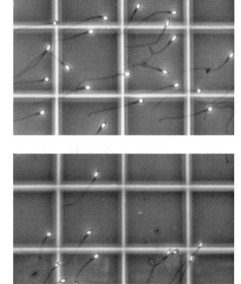

A semen analysis will determine whether a man's sperm count is in the healthy range (top), or whether it is poor (bottom).

Fertility tests for men Before performing any tests, a doctor will usually give a man a full examination to check for general signs of ill health or hormonal problems. The man's genitalia will also be checked for any obvious abnormality such as an undescended testis or signs of infection.

The main fertility test for men is semen analysis. This is when a freshly ejaculated specimen of semen is examined under a microscope. A man usually collects the specimen by masturbating into a special glass jar provided by his doctor and then elivers the specimen him self to the laboratory as soon as possible. To get an accurate report the semen should be examined within four hours of being ejaculated, so it is worth checking in advance when the laboratory can receive and examine a sample. Because sperm counts can vary enormously from day to day, two or three tests will usually be performed over a few weeks to get a true picture of a man's semen quality.

Foods that preserve male potency

A hardening of the arteries (atherosclerosis) not only causes heart disease by depriving the heart of its blood supply, it can also affect male fertility by preventing sufficient blood supply to the testes and penis, which can cause erectile problems and difficulties with sperm production. There are a number of self-help measures men can take to safeguard their sexual function and one of these is eating an artery-friendly diet. This involves reducing the intake of animal fats, for instance, by cutting down on meat and pastries and including the following:

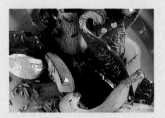

Eat five portions of vegetables or fruits a day. Try to vary the types you eat from week to week.

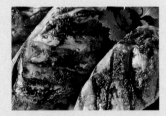

Instead of salt, flavour foods with herbs and spices, and choose sunflower or olive oil instead of butter.

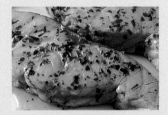

Include oily fish in your diet at least twice a week. Good choices include mackerel, salmon and herring.

A semen analysis will assess semen volume, the number of sperm, the motility of the sperm, and the proportion of normal healthy sperm present. The test will also determine whether the semen contains white blood cells or other signs of infection. The normal range for each of these measurements varies somewhat from one laboratory to another, so the results of this test will need to be discussed with your doctor.

Once the results of the semen analysis have been collected, further tests can be performed if necessary. A blood test, for example, will confirm the levels of testosterone, pituitary hormones and other hormone levels. If these are unusually low or high then your doctor will look for a cause, for example, low testosterone levels caused by high alcohol consumption (see chapter 8: Quitting Bad Habits) or high thyroxine levels as a result of an overactive thyroid (see page 171).

If an abnormality or a blockage in the sperm-producing system is suspected, a man may be referred to a urologist for x-rays, especially if there is a possibility that microsurgery can correct the fault.

Female fertility problems

In the past, fertility treatment tended to focus on the woman, not only because she was obviously the partner who failed to get pregnant, but also because this was the traditional domain of obstetricians and gynaecologists, who did not treat men at all. As a result, the causes of female fertility problems are better understood than those of men, and treatment for female infertility is better developed.

Ovulation disorders General health problems may disturb the hormonal balance between a woman's hypothalamus, her pituitary and her ovaries so that she fails to ovulate. This may lead to irregular or even absent periods. Low body weight, obesity, excessive exercise, emotional upset and thyroid problems can all disturb ovulation, so these should obviously be corrected before considering any fertility treatment. Usually, good health will restore ovulation in younger women affected by these problems. What's more, spontaneous pregnancy is likely to be safer and healthier for both mother and baby than if ovulation is induced while the woman is still in poor health.

On rare occasions the pituitary gland itself fails to send out the correct hormones because it is damaged or compressed by a tumour. In some instances, the ovaries may be unable to release any ova, for example, if the ovaries are damaged by severe endometriosis or polycystic ovarian syndrome (PCOS). Sometimes the ovaries age prematurely, in which case they have no more ova to release and will not respond to any treatment.

Testing for ovulation disorders Female hormones can also be measured by a blood test. Levels vary during the menstrual cycle, however, so it is important for the doctor to know exactly when you are menstruating. Levels of LH and FSH may be very high if the ovaries are not responding to the pituitary gland's outpouring of these hormones, as is the case during premature menopause. The ovaries may also be inhibited from releasing an ovum if high levels of prolactin from the pituitary are being released. This can occur if there is a pituitary tumour, during severe depression or stress, or you are breast-feeding (see Looking Ahead on page 50). Alternatively, hormone levels may be low if the hypothalamus or pituitary is failing, following weight loss, for example. If a woman has PCOS, her level of FSH may also be low.

A good test to determine whether you are ovulating or not is to measure levels of progesterone in the blood. Progesterone is only present in the second half of the menstrual cycle if you have ovulated. Ideally, progesterone levels should be measured seven days before your period as this is when they usually reach a peak. It is a good idea, therefore, to keep

DID YOU KNOW?

Having trouble conceiving is not just a modern dilemma. Although STDs have increased the number of fertility problems in recent years, there's always been a significant number of couples who could not get pregnant. In a fascinating study of English parish registers dated from 1550 to 1849, as many as one in ten marriages remained childless. Since it was at a time when contraception and safe abortion were not available, this was obviously not through choice. And where the woman was over 30 at the time of her marriage, the rate of childlessness was one in five.

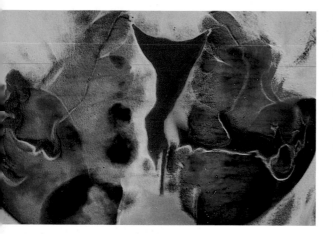

This hysterosalpin-gogram shows healthy, unblocked Fallopian tubes. The radio opaque dye is flowing freely up the uterus (centre) and through the Fallopian tubes to the ovaries on either side.

a careful record of your menstrual cycle. As it is common not to ovulate every month, this test should always be repeated if progesterone levels are low and don't seem to indicate ovulation. A temperature chart may also be used to determine whether you are ovulating (see pages 42–47).

Fertility problems arising from physical complications About 25 per cent of female fertility problems are caused by damage to the delicate Fallopian tubes that should provide transport and protection for the ovum, and later the newly fertilised zygote. Pelvic infection from sexually transmitted diseases or even appendicitis can cause scarring and blockage of these tubes. Severe endometriosis or scarring from abdominal surgery can also cause damage.

Perhaps another 15 per cent of female fertility problems are caused by abnormalities in the uterus or cervix, in which case a woman may conceive but later miscarry. Fibroids, for instance, distort the smooth shape of the uterus and may prevent the embryo implanting successfully. Infection in the endometrium can also lead to miscarriage. Sometimes, when a large cone of tissue has been taken from the cervix to treat early cancer, the cervix may not produce fertile mucus because of severe scarring (although such damage to the cervix is rare). Occasionally a woman may be born with an unusually shaped or double uterus that interferes with the smooth process of conception.

Examining the female pelvic organs Your doctor will examine you internally to feel if your uterus and ovaries are their normal size and shape. You should not feel any pain during this examination, and a very sensitive cervix or uterus may be a sign of infection. A vaginal speculum will also be inserted to view your cervix, allowing your doctor to take any swabs or a cervical smear as required.

For a more detailed examination of the size and shape of all your pelvic organs, a vaginal ultrasound scan can be performed. The blunt ultrasound probe sits in the vagina and gives a much better view of the lining of the uterus, the Fallopian tubes and the ovaries than an abdominal scan. However, to get a really detailed look at the pelvic organs, a laparoscopy is performed. This flexible telescope, with a fibre-optic light source, allows your gynaecologist to look directly inside your abdomen. Under general anaesthetic, a very small incision is made beneath the belly button and the laparoscope is gently inserted. To provide a good view, carbon dioxide gas is blown in through a needle inserted just at the pubic hairline, which inflates the abdomen. Simple operations, such as draining an ovarian cyst, can also be performed through a laparoscope.

The health of the Fallopian tubes is checked by a procedure known as a hysterosalpingography. In this procedure, radio opaque dye is injected through the cervix into the upper part of the uterus and x-rays are taken. The dye should pass right through the Fallopian tubes if they are not blocked (as semen should) and spill out near the ovaries. If the tubes have been blocked by disease, the dye will not flow. These x-rays give a view of the inside of the uterus, as well. The uterus can also by viewed directly by hysteroscopy, which is similar to laparoscopy except that the telescope is passed through the cervix. Laparoscopy and hysterosalpingography are often referred to as "lap and dye studies."

The postcoital test If a woman's cervical mucus is suspected of being infertile or hostile to sperm, a postcoital test can be conducted. At the presumed fertile time, a sample of cervical mucus is taken from the top of the woman's vagina a few hours after intercourse and examined under a microscope. Fertile mucus should show typical fern-like crystals, indicative of a high water content (see page 37). Sperm should also be seen swimming around and nurtured by the fertile mucus. These observations can be reassuring, but a poor test result may only indicate that it was not taken at the fertile time, in which case the test needs to be taken again. Poor sperm movement can be a sign of antisperm antibodies being produced by either partner. In these

TIME TO TALK
Counselling for IVF treatment

Before you and your partner consider fertility treatment you should be prepared for some of the emotional turmoil it can bring. Fertility clinics in the UK are legally required to provide counselling for couples contemplating treatment such as IVF, but you can start the ball rolling by considering the following issues with your partner:

• Will your relationship with your partner withstand the long periods of waiting and uncertainty that fertility treatment involves?

• How far are you prepared to go with investigation and treatment? Some couples find non-invasive treatment such as fertility drugs acceptable, but not assisted conception techniques such as IVF.

• If you decide to undergo IVF how will you feel about the "spare" embryos that are created, but not implanted in the uterus, and which are all potentially your children?

• Are you aware of the financial costs of infertility treatment? Remember, treatment may need to be repeated a few times before it is successful.

• If you both work, will you be able to take time off for appointments and treatment?

• How will you feel if treatment is unsuccessful? Will this be harder to bear than if you had never undergone treatment in the first place? Will you be able to strengthen your relationship with your partner if you can't have children?

instances, high dose steroid treatment may help the problem. Artificial insemination into the uterus and gamete intrafallopian transfer (GIFT: see page 186) may also help to overcome problems with anti-sperm antibodies.

Fertility treatment

It may seem obvious, but before a couple embarks on any course of fertility treatment, it's important that they undergo tests to establish the cause of their problem. All too often, couples are offered expensive, high-tech fertility treatments that have relatively low success rates when, in fact, the treatment may not be appropriate or the couple could conceive naturally with some simple improvements to their general health. However, if you and your doctor agree that fertility treatment is the best course of action, you can ask for a referral to a fertility clinic. These clinics offer a whole range of different treatments, depending on the cause of your difficulties.

Artificial insemination

This inexpensive and simple procedure involves semen being inserted into the top of the vagina or the uterus with a syringe. It helps couples when the problem lies in the man not being able to deposit sperm into the vagina, for example if the man has congenital abnormalities of the penis or suffers from retrograde ejaculation or impotence that makes intercourse impossible. It is also recommended when men have low sperm counts, women have hostile cervical mucus (artificially inseminated sperm can bypass the cervix) or when infertility is unexplained. When the husband's semen is used, the treatment is termed AIH (artificial insemination by husband). But the procedure can also be used with donor semen, for instance if the male partner cannot produce sufficient or healthy sperm, and in this case it is called AID (artificial insemination by donor).

TEST TUBE BABIES

In 1978 Louise Brown (seen below aged ten) became the first successful "test tube baby" to be born. Since then, tens of thousands of IVF babies have been born throughout the world. Overall, IVF babies do not seem to be at any increased risk of birth defects. However, because several embryos are usually transferred to the uterus to improve the chances of successful implantation, there is a higher risk of multiple pregnancy. This has associated health risks as well as large social repercussions.

Fertility drugs

If a woman has ovulation disorders that cannot be resolved with health improvements, such as correcting her exercise pattern or her body weight, fertility drugs can be given to stimulate ovum production. Drugs such as clomiphene, an antioestrogen, help to stimulate the natural

EATMENTS

Sunday

9pm

7960 342 431

BODY TREATMENTS

1 hr Pedicure - £16
(with exfoliation & massage)

Reshape & Varnish - £11

1 hr Manicure - £12
(with exfoliation & massage)

flow of hormones from the hypothalamus and pituitary to the ovary. Drugs that contain high levels of FSH and directly stimulate the ovary, such as human menopausal gonadotrophin, are more likely to produce multiple births than clomiphene because more than one ovum usually matures. A variety of other drugs act at different levels in the hypothalamic, pituitary and ovarian system and can all be used to treat ovulation disorders. The success of these fertility drugs depends on the man having normal, healthy sperm and the couple being able to have intercourse at the fertile time. Paradoxically, antioestrogens may inhibit fertile cervical mucus (one of the key fertility signals) and this can make it more difficult to detect a woman's most fertile time.

Surgery

If a woman has damaged Fallopian tubes, microsurgery can sometimes be performed to unblock them. Success depends not only on the skill of the surgeon, but also on the degree of damage. If the cilia are too damaged then the risk of an ectopic pregnancy increases. Where the surgery is unsuccessful, IVF (see below) can be offered, which bypasses tubal blockage. Surgery can also be offered to women who have single fibroids or small congenital abnormalities that prevent an embryo from implanting in the uterus.

Despite its fame and media coverage, IVF does not have a high success rate and should only be used when other ways to boost fertility have failed.

In vitro fertilisation (IVF)

Fertility problems arising from blocked or damaged Fallopian tubes, poor quality sperm, hostile cervical mucus, and unexplained causes may all be overcome using IVF. This is a technique where fertilisation takes place in a culture dish, bypassing the natural process of fertilisation in the Fallopian tubes ("in vitro" is Latin for "in glass"). Drugs are given to stimulate a woman's ovaries to produce several mature ova. The process is monitored by ultrasound and blood tests. When follicles develop sufficiently, the ova are collected by laparoscopy using a needle under ultrasound guidance. Meanwhile, her partner has to produce a semen sample, which is washed and from which the most healthy sperm are extracted. The sperm is mixed with the ova in a culture dish and observed under a microscope over the next two days. If an embryo or embryos develop, some of these can be placed into the woman's uterus using a fine tube slipped through the cervix. Blood tests over the next two weeks indicate if the

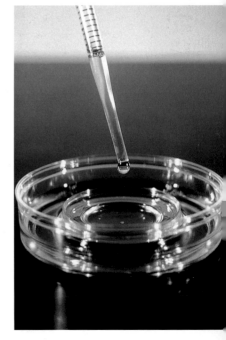

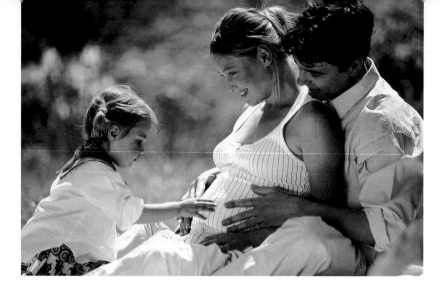

No one can guarantee a perfect baby – if such a thing exists – but you can be the best parents your child could hope for.

embryo has implanted. If fertilisation or implantation is unsuccessful, treatment can be repeated in another cycle. For some couples the treatment simply doesn't work, but younger couples with normal menstrual cycles and sperm counts are more likely to have success, as are those attending IVF clinics with sophisticated facilities and round the clock monitoring.

A simpler alternative to IVF, known as gamete intrafallopian transfer (GIFT), may sometimes be appropriate when the woman's tubes are not blocked and infertility is unexplained. GIFT involves placing ovum and sperm directly into the Fallopian tube to fertilise instead of in a culture dish, and some couples may prefer this option if they do not want the spare embryos that are created during IVF treatment.

Some closing thoughts on conception and parenthood

In trying to conceive and have a successful pregnancy, it's easy to lose sight of the object of all this planning and attention. The thought of becoming a parent is both exciting and daunting, but as you plan to conceive remember it is the child you must plan for, not just your pregnancy and the early days of babyhood. Although every parent longs for a healthy child, what every child longs for is to be loved, accepted and protected, whatever his or her personality, health, strengths and weaknesses may be.

USEFUL ADDRESSES

Action on Pre-Eclampsia (APEC)
84-88 Pinner Road, Harrow,
Middlesex HA1 4HZ
Helpline: 020 8427 3271
www.apec.org.uk

**Arthritis Research Campaign
(ARC)**
Copeman House, St Mary's Court,
St Mary's Gate,
Chesterfield S41 7TD
Tel: 01246 558033
www.arc.org.uk

**Association for Improvements in
the Maternity Services**
5 St Ann's Court, Grove Road,
Surbiton, Surrey KT6 4BE
Tel: 0870 765 1433
www.aims.org.uk

Association for Post-Natal Illness
145 Dawes Road,
London SW6 7EB
Tel: 020 7386 0868
www.apni.org

**British Association of Cancer
United Patients (BACUP)**
3 Bath Place, Rivington Street,
London EC2A 3DR
Information line: 0808 800 1234
www.cancerbacup.org.uk

British Diabetic Association
10 Queen Anne Street,
London W1M 0DB
Tel: 020 7424 1000

Cystic Fibrosis Trust
11 London Road, Bromley,
Kent BR1 1BY
Tel: 020 8464 7211
www.cftrust.org.uk

Down's Syndrome Association
155 Mitcham Road,
London SW17 9PG
Tel: 020 8682 4001
www.downs-syndrome.org.uk

Fertility UK
Bury Knowle Health Centre,
207 London Road, Headington,
Oxford OX3 9JA
www.fertility.uk.org

Foresight Association
28 The Paddock, Godalming,
Surrey GU7 1XD
Tel: 01483 427839
www.foresight-preconception.org.uk

fpa (Family Planning Association)
2-12 Pentonville Road,
London N1 9FP
Tel: 0845 310 1334
www.fpa.org.uk

The Impotence Association
PO Box 10296,
London SW17 9WH
Helpline: 020 8767 7791
www.impotence.org.uk

**Issue (National Infertility
Association)**
114 Lichfield Street,
Walsall WS1 1FZ
Tel: 01922 722888
www.issue.co.uk

Iyengar Yoga Institute
223A Randolph Avenue,
London W9 1NL
Tel: 020 7624 3080
www.iyi.org.uk

The Maternity Alliance
45 Beech Street,
London EC2P 2LX
Tel: 020 7588 8582
www.maternityalliance.org.uk

The Miscarriage Association
Clayton Hospital, Northgate,
Wakefield,
West Yorkshire WF1 3JS
Tel: 01924 200795
www.miscarriageassociation.org.uk

The Multiple Sclerosis Society
25 Effie Road,
London SW5 1EE
24 hour helpline: 0800 800 0800
www.mssociety.org.uk

National Asthma Campaign
Providence House,
Providence Place,
London N1 0NT
Tel: 020 7226 2260
Helpline: 08457 010203
www.asthma.org.uk

National Childbirth Trust
Alexandra House,
Oldham Terrace,
London W3 6NH
Tel: 0870 4448707
www.nctpregnancyandbabycare.com

National Eczema Society
Hill House, Highgate Hill,
London N19 5NA
Tel: 020 7281 3553
Helpline: 0870 2413604
www.eczema.org

**The National
Endometriosis Society**
50 Westminster Palace Gardens
1-7 Artillery Row,
London SW1P 1RL
Tel: 020 7222 2776
www.endo.org.uk

**National Radiological
Protection Board**
Chilton, Didcot,
Oxon OX11 0RQ
Tel: 01235 831600
www.nrpb.org.uk

**Society of Teachers of the
Alexander Technique**
1st Floor, Linton House,
39-51 Highgate Road,
London NW5 1RS
Tel: 020 7284 3338
www.stat.org.uk

INDEX

ACKNOWLEDGEMENTS

PICTURE CREDITS

Front jacket Ace Photo Agency (top & centre), Telegraph Colour library (bottom); **6** Tony Stone Images; **7** The Stock Market; **8-9** Tony Stone Images; **10** Images Colour Library; **12** (top) Prof. P. Motta/Dept of Anatomy/University 'La Sapienza', Rome/SPL, (left) SPL, (right) Prof. P. M. Motta, G. Macchiarelli, S.A. Nottolal/SPL; **16** Prof. Motta/Dept of Anatomy/University 'La Sapienza', Rome/SPL; **18** The Stock Market; **19** Mehau Kulyk/SPL; **20** CNRI/SPL; **21** CNRI/SPL; **24** D. Phillips/SPL; **25** Linda Lewis c/o Frank Lane Picture Library; **26** Andy Walker/Midland Fertility Services/SPL; **29** National Medical Slide Library, London; **30** Angela Hampton/Family Life Pictures; **31** Tony Stone Images; **35** Images Colour Library; **36** Tony Stone Images; **37** Dr. Caroline Finlayson/Mr. Paul Carter, St.George's Hospital, London; **40** Tony Stone Images; **45** The Stock Market; **48** Images Colour Library; **50** Tony Stone Images; **52-53** The Stock Market; **54** Collections/Sandra Lousada; **55** Collection of Israel Antiquities Authority. Exhibited at and photographed by the Israel Museum; **56** Images Colour Library; **57** Angela Hampton/Family Life Pictures; **59** The Stock Market; **60** CNRI/SPL; **62** Tony Stone Images; **63** Angela Hampton /Family Life Pictures; **64** Images Colour Library; **68** Images Colour Library; **71** The Stock Market; **72** Tony Stone Images; **74** Ruth Jenkinson/Mother and Baby Picture Library; **80** Tony Stone Images; **84, 173** Images Colour Library; **89** Telegraph Colour Library; **90** Profs P. M. Motta and S.Correr/SPL; **96** Museo Correr, Venice, Italy/ Giraudon/Bridgeman Art Library, London; **99** The Stock Market; **100** (top) Tony Stone Images; **104** Tony Stone Images; **110** Tony Stone Images; **114** Sidney Moulds/SPL; **116** Image Bank; **117** Angela Hampton/Family Life Pictures; **119** Tony Stone Images; **120** Tony Stone Images; **123** Eye Ubiquitous; **124** Pictor International; **127** Image Bank; **128** Tony Stone Images; **129** Tony Stone Images; **131** National Library of Medicine/SPL; **133** Tony Stone Images; **136** Angela Hampton/Family Life Pictures; **137** The Stock Market; **138** The Stock Market; **141** Rosenfeld Images Ltd/SPL; **142** Telegraph Colour Library; **144** Telegraph Colour Library; **146** Tony Stone Images; **147** The Stock Market; **150** Ecoscene/Chris Knapton; **152** Image Bank; **154** Profs P. M. Motta and S. Makabe/SPL; **163** CC Studio/SPL; **165** Tony Stone Images; **167** Tony Stone Images; **172** Tony Stone Images; **176** Tony Stone Images; **174-175** Tony Stone Images; **177** Simon Fraser/SPL; **179** James King-Holmes/SPL; **182** CNRI/SPL; **184** Rex Features; **185** Hank Morgan/SPL **186** Tony Stone Images.

ILLUSTRATIONS

Kathy Wyatt, anatomical illustrations.

CARROLL & BROWN ACKNOWLEDGEMENTS

We would very much like to thank the following people for their assistance in the making of this book:

Professor John Thomas Queenan from the School of Medicine, Department of Obstetrics and Gynecology at Georgetown University Medical Center, and Jane Knight from Fertility UK for additional medical advice; Sandra Schneider for picture research; Madeline Weston for indexing; Betsy Hosegood for proofreading; Rachel Goldsmith, Finn Lewis, Kenta Namba and Jane Felstead for additional design assistance; Dawn Henderson for additional editorial assistance; Kym Menzies, Jessamina Owens, and Bettina Graham for hair and make-up; Colin Tatham for photographic assistance; and Poppy Body for home economy.